Traditional Processing and Modern Studies

传统中药炮制与现代研究
汉英对照

主 编 钟凌云 杨 明
Editor-in-Chief Lingyun Zhong Ming Yang

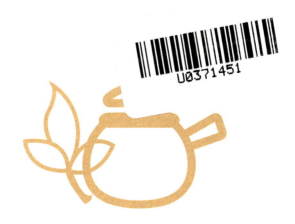

全国百佳图书出版单位
中国中医药出版社
·北 京·

图书在版编目（CIP）数据

传统中药炮制与现代研究：汉英对照/钟凌云，杨明主编.—北京：中国中医药出版社，2021.11
ISBN 978-7-5132-7155-4

Ⅰ.①传… Ⅱ.①钟…②杨… Ⅲ.①中药炮制学—研究—汉、英 Ⅳ.① R283

中国版本图书馆 CIP 数据核字（2021）第 173846 号

中国中医药出版社出版
北京经济技术开发区科创十三街 31 号院二区 8 号楼
邮政编码　100176
传真　010-64405721
廊坊市晶艺印务有限公司印刷
各地新华书店经销

开本 787×1092　1/16　印张 21.5　字数 373 千字
2021 年 11 月第 1 版　2021 年 11 月第 1 次印刷
书号　ISBN 978-7-5132-7155-4

定价　68.80 元
网址　www.cptcm.com

服 务 热 线　010-64405510
购 书 热 线　010-89535836
维 权 打 假　010-64405753

微信服务号　zgzyycbs
微商城网址　https://kdt.im/LIdUGr
官方微博　http://e.weibo.com/cptcm
天猫旗舰店网址　https://zgzyycbs.tmall.com

如有印装质量问题请与本社出版部联系（010-64405510）
版权专有　侵权必究

《传统中药炮制与现代研究：汉英对照》
编 委 会

主　审	龚千锋	**Presiding judge**　　QianFeng Gong
主　编	钟凌云　杨　明	**Editor-in-Chief**　　Lingyun Zhong　Ming Yang
副主编	叶喜德　祝　婧	**Deputy Editors**　　Xide Ye　Jing Zhu

编　委（按姓氏笔画排序）　　**Editorial board**

于　欢（江西中医药大学）　　Huan Yu (Jiangxi University of Chinese Medicine)

于晓敏（温州医科大学）　　Xiaomin Yu (Wenzhou Medical University)

万莉莉（江西中医药大学）　　Lili Wan (Jiangxi University of Chinese Medicine)

王艳霓（江西省德安县中医院）　　Yanni Wang (Jiangxi De'an Chinese Medicine Hospital)

吕心欢（北京中医药大学）　　Xinhuan Lv (Beijing University of Chinese Medicine)

李晓芳（江西中医药大学附属医院）　　Li Xiaofang (The Affiliated Hospital of Jiangxi University of TCM)

陈　浩（江西中医药大学附属医院）　　Chen Hao (The Affiliated Hospital of Jiangxi University of TCM)

欧阳辉（江西中医药大学）　　Hui Ouyang (Jiangxi University of Chinese Medicine)

黄　艺（江西中医药大学）　　Yi Huang (Jiangxi University of Chinese Medicine)

童恒力（江西中医药大学）　　Tong Hengli (Jiangxi University of Chinesse Medicine)

颜干明（江西继中堂健康科技有限公司）　　Yan ganming (Jiangxi Jizhongtang Health Technology Co. Ltd)

前 言

中药炮制是中国历史上的珍贵遗产,根据中医药相关专业学习要求及继承和发展这一珍贵遗产的需要,由钟凌云、杨明教授主编的《传统炮制与现代研究》汉英对照一书,突出学科教育的前沿性,使中药炮制学科能更好地走向国际化,便于国内外学者了解中药炮制学科发展情况。该书以传统炮制与现代研究为编写内容,在注重传统理论和方法的同时,紧扣现代研究成果,采用汉英双语形式编写,内容兼顾其他学科,以确保知识的完整性。

全书分为三部分:第一部分"绪论"、第二部分"传统炮制"、第三部分"现代研究"。绪论概括本书内容提纲。第二部分"传统炮制"围绕江西"樟""建"两帮及其他炮制流派的发展脉络和形成特色,对炮制流派涉及的主要炮制方法和工具等进行了描述。对炮制工具配有图文,使其更加直观,增加读者的感性认识。就传统炮制方法,探讨了其对现代中药炮制发展的启示。第三部分"现代研究"主要从炮制机理、炮制工艺、炮制前后成分、药效和质量标准等方面,对中药炮制现代研究进行了阐述。编者以实例形式,增加了他们从事中药炮制研究的部分内容,以加深读者的理解,并对该学科未来发展进行了展望。中文部分的参考文献,英文部分略。

· PREFACE ·

    Traditional Chinese medicine processing (TCMP) is a precious heritage in the history of China. Under the learning requirements of majors related to Chinese medicine as well as the needs of inheritance and development of TCMP. *Traditional Processing and Modern Studies* is a bilingual monograph written and edited in Chinese and English by Lingyun Zhong. It highlights the frontiers of this subject for a better internationalization, including facilitating the understanding of the subject development of TCMP around domestic and foreign scholars. This book is written based on traditional medicine processing and modern research. Focusing on ancient theories and methods, where modern research results are closely followed. The content also considers additional subjects which safeguard the integrity of knowledge.

    In general, the full text of this book is divided into three sections: part I, part II and part III. The part I outlines the contents of the monograph. While the part II focuses on the traditional processing, which reflects the development and characteristics of Zhang Society and Jian Society of Jiangxi along with other TCMP schools, it describes the main processing methods and tools involved in different processing schools. The monograph offers the illustrations of processing tools to make them more intuitive and improve the reader's perceptual knowledge. Concerning the traditional processing method, its enlightenment to the development of modern Chinese medicine processing is discussed. Finally, the last part of the monograph is modern research. The modern research of TCMP is mainly expounded on the aspects of processing mechanism, processing technology, composition before and after processing, efficacy, and quality standards. The editors shared their experiences on the processing of traditional Chinese medicine for the reader's better understanding and provided their prospects for future development of this subject. We keep the references as the original version only in Chinese.

    The distinctive feature of this book is that it is the effective fusion between TCMP tra-

本书内容的主要特点是：把中药炮制传统与现代研究内容进行了有效融合，借助实例形式，采用双语文字编写，使本书内容不仅创新，而且更具时效性，可为从事中药炮制行业的从业人员及国际学员学习提供参考。通过中药、化学、炮制、语言等多学科交叉互融，揭示了中药炮制的科学内涵，丰富和发展了炮制理论，也为中药炮制学科走向国际化，打下良好基础。

本书在编写过程中，得到参编单位及相关专家的大力支持和指导，在此深表感谢！

编写过程中难免有不足和错漏之处，恳请各院校同行和读者，在使用过程中提出宝贵意见，以便进一步完善。

编者

2021年3月10日

dition and modern research content. With the help of examples and bilingual literature, the content of this book is not only innovative but also more time-effective. References could be provided for both industry practitioners and international students engaged in the processing of traditional Chinese medicine. Through the interdisciplinary integration of basic knowledge of traditional Chinese medicine, chemistry, processing, and language, the scientific connotation of TCMP is revealed, and the processing theory is enrichingly developed. Besides, it lays a good foundation for the internationalization of TCMP.

In the process of compiling, we have received strong support and guidance from the participating units and relevant experts. Thank you very much!

There are inevitably shortcomings and omissions. I urge colleagues and readers of various institutions to put forward your valuable opinions in the process of using this monograph for further improvements and modifications.

Writers
Mar 10, 2021

目 录

第一部分 绪 论 ·· 001
一、中药炮制的定义和性质 ··· 002
二、中药炮制的起源和发展 ··· 006
三、中药炮制的法规 ·· 006

第二部分 传统炮制 ·· 011

第一章 传统炮制流派发展概况 ·· 012
一、樟帮的起源和发展 ·· 012
二、建昌帮的起源和发展 ·· 014
三、川帮的起源和发展 ·· 016
四、京帮的起源和发展 ·· 018

第二章 各流派的炮制特点 ·· 022
一、樟帮的炮制特点 ·· 022
二、建昌帮的炮制特点 ·· 028
三、川帮的炮制特点 ·· 034
四、京帮的炮制特点 ·· 036
五、各流派炮制特点比较 ·· 038

第三章 主要常用炮制方法 ·· 046
一、净选加工 ·· 046
二、饮片切制 ·· 054
三、炒法 ·· 062
四、炙法 ·· 070
五、煅法 ·· 084
六、蒸煮焯法 ·· 088
七、其他方法 ·· 092

· CATALOG ·

Part I Introduction ... 001

    Section One   The Definition and Nature of Processing of Chinese Herbal Medicine (PCHM) ... 003

    Section Two   Origination and Development of PCHM ... 007

    Section Three   Laws and Regulations of PCHM ... 007

Part II Traditional Processing of Chinese Herbal Medicine ... 011

Chapter One   Summary of the Development of Traditional Schools of PCHM ... 013

    Section One   The Origin and Development of Zhang Society ... 013

    Section Two   The Origin and Development of Jianchang Society ... 015

    Section Three   The Origin and Development of Chuan Society ... 017

    Section Four   The Origin and Development of Jing Society ... 019

Chapter Two   Processing Characteristics of Different Schools of PCHM ... 023

    Section One   Processing Technology Characteristics of Zhang Society ... 023

    Section Two   Processing Technology Characteristics of Jianchang Society ... 029

    Section Three   Processing Technology Characteristics of Chuan Society ... 035

    Section Four   Processing Technology Characteristics of Jing Society ... 037

    Section Five   Comparison of Processing Characteristics of Different Schools ... 039

Chapter Three   Main Processing Technology ... 047

    Section One   Cleansing ... 047

    Section Two   Cutting of Prepared Drugs in Pieces ... 055

    Section Three   Stir-frying ... 063

    Section Four   Stir-frying with Liquid Adjuvant Material ... 071

    Section Five   Calcining Method ... 085

    Section Six   Steaming, Boiling, and Blanching ... 089

    Section Seven   Other Ways ... 093

第四章　传统炮制技术工具 ······ 108
　　一、净制工具 ······ 108
　　二、切制工具 ······ 128
　　三、炒制工具 ······ 168
　　四、蒸煮制工具 ······ 180
　　五、煅制工具 ······ 182
　　六、其他制法工具 ······ 188
　　七、干燥工具 ······ 194

第三部分　现代研究 ······ 203

第五章　炮制的现代研究概况 ······ 204
　　一、概述 ······ 204
　　二、中药炮制研究的内容 ······ 208
　　三、中药炮制研究的方法 ······ 224

第六章　现代研究主要技术与方法 ······ 250
　　一、新工艺技术的应用 ······ 250
　　二、代谢组学 ······ 254
　　三、药代动力学 ······ 256
　　四、组分结构理论 ······ 260
　　五、分子生物学技术 ······ 264

第七章　对炮制成分和药效变化的现代研究 ······ 272
　　一、炮制对化学成分变化的影响 ······ 274
　　二、炮制对中药药理作用的影响 ······ 280

第八章　研究实例 ······ 290
　　实例一　青黛炮制过程各环节原理的系统研究 ······ 290
　　实例二　基于传质、传热规律的传统的干馏蛋黄油炮制研究 ······ 292
　　实例三　鳖血柴胡炮制工艺与机制研究 ······ 292
　　实例四　基于药辅合一的药汁制法炮制研究 ······ 294

Chapter Four Traditional Processing Technology Tools ············ 109

Section One　Cleaning Tools ············ 109

Section Two　Cutting Tools ············ 129

Section Three　Frying Tools ············ 169

Section Four　Steaming and Boiling Tools ············ 181

Section Five　Forging tools ············ 183

Section Six　Other Tools of Processing ············ 189

Section Seven　Dry Tools ············ 195

Part III Modern Research of PCHM ············ 203

Chapter Five The Introduction of Modern Research of PCHM ············ 205

Section One　The Summary ············ 205

Section Two　Research on the PCHM ············ 209

Section Three　The Methods of PCHM Research ············ 225

Chapter Six Main Techniques and Methods of Modern Research of PCHM ············ 251

Section One　The Application of New Process Technology ············ 251

Section Two　Metabolomics ············ 255

Section Three　Pharmacokinetics ············ 257

Section Four　Component Structure Theory ············ 261

Section Five　Molecular Biology ············ 265

Chapter Seven Modern Research on the Changes of Contents and Pharmacological Effects Before and After PCHM ············ 273

Section One　Effect on the Changes of Chemical Composition by Processing ············ 275

Section Twenty　Effect of Processing on Pharmacological Action of Traditional Chinese Medicine ············ 281

Chapter Eight Examples of Modern Research of PCHM ············ 291

Example 1　Systematical Research of Processing Mechanism During Every Step in Processing of Indigo Naturalis ············ 291

Example 2　The Study on Processing of Traditional Distilled Egg Yolk Oil Based on the Rules of Mass Transfer and Heat Transfer ············ 293

Example 3　The Study on Processing Method and Mechanism of Bupleuri Radix Stir-fried with Turtle Blood ············ 293

Example 4　The Study on Medicine Juice Process Based on Rules of Drugs plus Supplement ············ 295

实例五　天南星科有毒中药矾制解毒的共性规律研究 ·················· 296

　　实例六　基于"析霜"特色的江西姜厚朴减毒增效炮制机制研究 ·················· 298

　　实例七　"盐炙入肾－肾主骨"的物质基础和作用机制研究 ·················· 300

　　实例八　基于栀子"炒炭存性"的科学内涵探究 ·················· 302

　　实例九　基于"寒热药性变化"的黄连炮制研究 ·················· 304

　　实例十　基于多种热力学形态水火共制熟三七炮制研究 ·················· 304

　　实例十一　江西特色蜜麸枳壳减燥增效炮制机制研究 ·················· 306

　　实例十二　传统炆制黄精的现代研究 ·················· 306

　　实例十三　基于多物料、多流程的传统炮附子炮制研究 ·················· 308

　　实例十四　基于UHP-MS/MS和化学分析法对天麻炮制品中的主成分分析 ·················· 310

　　实例十五　药代/毒代动力学技术在中药炮制现代研究中的应用 ·················· 312

第九章　现代炮制研究展望 ·················· 314

　　一、药材产地初加工、饮片炮制真正做到工艺规范化、规模化、
　　　　产业化和一体化 ·················· 316

　　二、充分利用现代先进科技手段，真正做到传承与发展有机结合，进一步
　　　　推进质量控制标准化、统一化 ·················· 320

Example 5　The Study on Common Regulation of Detoxification of Toxic Chinese Medical Herbs in
　　　　　　Araceaen Processed with Alummen ··· 297
Example 6　The Study on Processing Mechanism of Detoxification and Synergism of Magnoliae
　　　　　　Officinalis Cortex Processed with Ginger Juice with Method Record in Zhangshu Branch
　　　　　　in Jiangxi province Based on the Character of Frost Formation ···························· 299
Example 7　The Substances and Mechanism Study on 'Salt Roasting into Kidney-the Kidney
　　　　　　Being in Charge of Bone' ··· 301
Example 8　The Scientific Connotation Study on 'Carbonizing by Stir-frying with Function
　　　　　　Preserve' of Gareniae Fructus ··· 303
Example 9　The Study on Processing of Goptidis Rhizoma Based on the Theory of 'Changes
　　　　　　of Cold and Hot Properties' ··· 305
Example 10　The Study on Processed Notoginseng Radix Et Rhizoma Based on Hydrothermal
　　　　　　　Copolymerization of Various Thermodynamic Forms ·· 305
Example 11　The Study on Processing Mechanism of Reduce Dryness and Increase Efficiency of
　　　　　　　Honey-Bran Stir-fried Auranii Fructus with Jiangxi Processing Character ···················· 307
Example 12　The Modern Study on Processing of Traditional Simmering Polygonati Rhizoma ········ 307
Example 13　The Study on Traditional Blast-fried Aconiti Lateralis Radix Praeparata Based on
　　　　　　　Multiple Supplements and Steps ·· 309
Example 14　Identification and Characterization of Key Chemical Constituents in Processed
　　　　　　　Gastrodiae Rhizoma Using UHPLC-MS/MS and Chemometric Methods ···················· 311
Example 15　The Application of Pharmacokinetics and Toxicokinetics in Modern Research of
　　　　　　　Chinese Medicine Herbs Processing ·· 313

Chapter Nine　Research Outlook of PCHM ·· 315
　Section One　Roughly Processed CMM and the Processing of Herbal Slices Should be Truly
　　　　　　　　Standardized, Scaled, Industrialized and Integrated. ··· 317
　Section Two　Make Full Use of Modern Advanced Scientific Technology to Achieve the True
　　　　　　　　Combination of Inheritance and Development, and Further Promote the
　　　　　　　　Standardization and Unification of Quality Control ··· 321

Part I
第一部分

绪论
Introduction

中药炮制是什么？中药炮制的科学原理是什么？当接触这门古老而又年轻的学科时，首先应理解中药炮制的作用，其前提就是了解何为中药炮制。

一、中药炮制的定义和性质

1. 定义

（1）中药炮制的定义：根据中医药理论，按照辨证用药的需要和药物自身的性质，以及调剂制剂不同要求所采取的一项制药技术，即为中药炮制。广义包括净制、切制和炮制；狭义包括炒、炙、煅、蒸、煮、燀、复制、发酵、发芽、制霜、烘焙、水飞等。

（2）中药炮制学的定义：中药炮制学是专门研究中药炮制理论、工艺、规格标准、历史沿革及其发展的学科。

（3）关于中药炮制理论：阐明炮制原理，例如药物炒炭后增强其止血作用，中医理论认为，"红见黑则止"（五行相克理论中水克火，而黑属水，红属火）。而现代理论则认为，药物炒炭后能增加鞣质含量，从而增加血中的钙、铁离子含量，可促进血凝。

（4）关于工艺方面：目的在于提高炮制作用并规范炮制工艺。例如马钱子，有砂炒、油炸、尿泡、醋制，其中尿泡为江西樟帮的特色制法，炮制工艺研究的目的是保存药效的同时对传统工艺进行改进研究。

第一部分 绪 论

Part I Introduction

What is the meaning of the Processing of Chinese Herbal Medicine (PCHM)? And what is the scientific principle of PCHM? When coming into contact with this ancient and young subject, you should first understand the role of PCHM, and the premise is to understand what Traditional Chinese Medicine (TCM) is.

Section One　The Definition and Nature of Processing of Chinese Herbal Medicine (PCHM)

1. Definition

(1) The definition of PCHM: According to TCM theory, PCHM refers to a kind of pharmaceutical technology, which is following the medication differentiation needs, the nature of the drug itself, and the different requirements for compounding. Broadly speaking, the contents of PCHM includes cleansing, cutting, and processing. In a narrow sense, the contents of PCHM cover frying, stir-frying, calcining, steaming, boiling, blanching, repeated processing, fermentating, sprouting, frost-like powder making, baking, grinding in water, etc.

(2) The definition of subject of PCHM: The Subject of PCHM refers to the subject specializing in the theory, technology, specification standard, history, and development of PCHM.

(3) About the theory of PCHM: It mainly refers to clarify the scientific connotation of theories and the mechanism of processing. For example, carbonizing drugs by stir-frying could enhance the hemostatic effect of the drug. The TCM theory holds that "when red blood meets with black drugs, bleeding stops"(The five elements promote and constrain mutually：metal-wood-water-fire-earth). Modern studies show that carbonizing drugs by stir-frying could increase the content of tannin, increase calcium and iron ion content in blood, and promoting blood coagulation.

(4) About the technology of PCHM: The purpose to study the technology of PCHM is to enhance the efficiency of processing and to standardize the processing technology. Taking Strychni Semen (Maqianzi) as an example, there are several methods, such as stir-frying with sand technology, frying with oil technology, soaking in urine technology, and processing with vinegar technology which are applied to processing Strychni Semen. Among them, soaking in urine technology is considered the best method to relived the toxicity and enhance the effect of the drug. But considering the assistant of urine is unaccepted by normal people, finding the replacement of urine assistant and regular processing technology is necessary.

（5）有关规格标准：目的在于规范饮片类型、规格和质量标准。包括饮片的片型、厚薄、外观色泽及成分含量等，以此确定中药饮片的质量标准，如巴豆霜，《中华人民共和国药典》（下文简称《中国药典》）规定其含脂肪油量在18%～20%之间，马钱子的炮制以士的宁含量作为指标，从而使中药饮片质量稳定可控具有可操作性，克服经验判断的局限性。

2. 中药炮制学的基本任务

（1）探讨炮制原理：炮制原理是指药物炮制的科学依据，探讨在一定工艺条件下，中药在炮制过程中产生的物理变化和化学变化，以及因这些变化而产生的药理作用的改变和这些改变所产生的临床意义。它包括对中药炮制减毒、增强疗效、缓和药性、产生新药效的原理研究等内容。例如对于黑豆汁蒸何首乌、醋制延胡索的炮制机制研究等。

（2）改进炮制工艺：可从两方面来理解，首先是对传统炮制工艺的改进，如泽泻，从古至今都采用盐炙法进行炮制，但现代研究证明，盐炙泽泻的功效与其他非盐制炮制工艺无显著区别，因此，认为泽泻盐炙还有待于进一步商榷。其次，对传统炮制工艺从经验判别转为数据化的工艺参数，也是对炮制工艺进行改进的一方面，是实现饮片工业化和规模化的必然趋势。

（3）制定饮片质量标准：饮片的质量标准包括外观鉴别（如色泽、气味等）和内在质量判别，如饮片的有效成分含量、有毒成分限量、农药残留量、重金属含量及指纹图谱、特征图谱等。

3. 中药炮制学与其他学科的关系

（1）与传统中医药理论的关系：中药炮制是在中医药理论指导下进行的制药技术。

（2）与中药化学的关系：通过炮制会改变药物的化学成分，因此，须要掌握中药化学的基本知识，以此了解药物的主要成分在炮制前后可能会发生的变化，如含生物碱类成分的黄柏，其中的小檗碱易溶于水，因此，在用水处理黄柏时，要采用"抢水洗"的方式，避免有效成分小檗碱的损失。

Part I Introduction

(5) About the specification standards of PCHM: The main purpose is to standardize the types, specifications, and quality standard of processed drugs in decoction pieces. The shape, thickness of the slices, the color, and the contents of the components of slices help set the quality standards of the processed products. For example, in the *Pharmacopoeia of the People's Republic of China* (the *Chinese Pharmacopoeia* in short), the contents of fat oil in Crotonis Fructus should be contained between 18% to 20% . The content of strychnine is also the indicator to control the quality of the processed Strychni Semen, All the index of slices mentioned above are applied to make the quality controllable, so as to overcome limitations of empirical discrimination.

2. The basic task of PCHM

(1) Exploring the principle of PCHM: The principle of PCHM refers to the scientific basis of PCHM, which discuss the physical and chemical change of drugs, and thus the changes of pharmacopeia and clinical use with drugs' processing, including the mechanism of reducing toxicity, enhancing the effect, and producing new effects. For example, the study of the processing mechanism of Polygoni Multiflori Radix (Heshouwu) steamed with black bean juice, Corydalis Rhizoma (Yanhusuo) stir-fried with vinegar, etc.

(2) Technology improvement of PCHM: The improvement of the PCHM technology includes two aspects. Firstly, to improve the traditional processing technology, such as Alismatis Rhizoma (Zexie), which is processed with salt since ancient times, but modern research showed that the effect of processing with salt had no significant difference from processing without salt, the technology of processing Rhizoma Alismatis with salt need further study. Secondly, transfer the traditional processing technology from empirical discrimination to digital processing parameters, is also the other aspect of improvement of technology of processing, which is the inevitable trend of realizing the industrialization and mass production of prepared slices.

(3) Formulate quality standard of prepared slices: The quality standard of prepared slices includes the identification of appearance (such as color, smell, etc.) and intrinsic quality judgment, such as the content of effective components, the limit of toxic components, pesticide residues, heavy metal contents, and fingerprint spectrum, Characteristic Atlas, etc.

3. Relationship between PCHM and other subjects

(1) Relationship between PCHM and the theory of TCM: The PCHM is the pharmaceutical technologies conducted under the direction of the TCM theories.

(2) Relationship between PCHM and Chemistry of Chinese Materia Medica: The components in drugs would be changed through processing, it is necessary to grasp the basic knowledge of Chemistry of Chinese Materia Medica to know the change of the main component in drugs after processing. For example, the alkaloid components exist in some drugs, such as Phellodendri Chinensis Cortex (Huangbai), the affective component of berberine in Phellodendri Chinensis Cortex (Huangbai) is easily resolved in water. In avoiding the loss of berberine, when processing this drug with water (wash, softening, and so on), it is better to process it in water as short as possible.

（3）与分析化学的关系：分析化学包括两方面，化学分析和仪器分析。在化学分析方面，对药物的生熟制品进行化学分析，通过定性定量来判断孰优孰劣。在仪器分析方面，须要掌握高效液相色谱、气相色谱、质谱、紫外光谱、红外光谱等仪器设备的使用，以便更好地分析炮制前后成分的变化规律。

（4）与中药鉴定学的关系：可通过掌握鉴定学知识，对药物切制成饮片之后的饮片断面进行鉴定，判别真伪优劣。

二、中药炮制的起源和发展

1. 中药炮制的起源

中药炮制起源于原始社会，随着中药的发现而发展，并与火的发明、烹饪技术的发展密切相关（包括辅料和贮存器的发展）。

2. 中药炮制的发展

中药炮制发展经历了四个阶段，中药炮制技术的起始和形成时期（汉以前）；炮制理论的形成时期（金元明时期）；炮制品种和技术的扩大应用时期（清代）；炮制振兴、发展时期（中华人民共和国成立后）。

三、中药炮制的法规

2001年12月颁布的中华人民共和国药品管理法，是目前药品生产、使用、检验的基本法律，这便是中药炮制所必须遵守的法规。

《中国药典》是炮制所要遵循的国家级法规，附录设有"中药炮制通则"专篇，规定了各种炮制方法的定义、具有共性的操作方法及质量要求，是属国家级饮片质量标准。

《全国中药炮制规范》由原卫生部药政局组织编撰，于1988年出版，作为部级中药饮片炮制标准（暂行），附录中收录了"中药炮制通则"及"全国中药炮制法概况表"等。

(3) Relationship between PCHM and analytical chemistry: This relationship includes two aspects, chemical analysis, and instrumental analysis. For the aspect of chemical analysis, it is necessary to know about the qualitative and quantitative change of components through chemical analysis; For aspect of instrumental analysis, the methods of instrument use, such as HPLC, LC, MS, UV, IR, should be understood to analysis the change regulation of components before and after processing.

(4) Relationship between PCHM and identification of Chinese Materia Medica: The knowledge of identification of Chinese Materia Medica could be used to discriminate the true or false, good or bad of the drug through the cross-section of prepared slices.

Section Two   Origination and Development of PCHM

1. Origination of PCHM

The PCHM was originated in primitive society, developed with the discovery of the Chinese Materia Medica, the invention of fire, and the development of cooking technology (including the development of food assistant and food storage).

2. Development of PCHM

The development of PCHM went through four stages, namely, the origination and formation period of PCHM technology (before the Han Dynasty), the formation period of processing theory (Jin, Yuan, and Ming Dynasties), the expanding application period of processing varieties and technology (Qing Dynasty), the rejuvenation and development period of processing (since the founding of the People's Republic of China).

Section Three   Laws and Regulations of PCHM

The Drug Administration Law of the People's Republic of China (PRC) promulgated in December 2001 is the basic law for the production, use, and inspection of pharmaceuticals. This is the law that must be observed in PCHM.

Chinese Pharmacopoeia is considered the national regulations of PCHM. The appendix in the pharmacopeia contains the "General Principles of Chinese Medicine Processing", which stipulates the definitions of various processing technologies, common technique operation methods, and quality requirements. It is the national level standard for prepared slices.

The *National Chinese Herb Medicine Processing Regulations* was compiled by the China Academy of Chinese Medical Sciences published in 1988. It is the ministerial level standard for prepared slices. The appendix there contains "General Rules of the Processing of Chinese Herbal Medicine" and "Overview of the National Processing of Chinese Herbal Medicine Methods" etc.

对于地方中药饮片标准，只有在国家与部级标准中没有收载此品种的情况下，才能制定适合本地的标准，同时应当报国务院药品监督管理部门备案，如《江西省中药炮制规范》《福建省中药炮制规范》等。

For the local standards of prepared slices, only under the circumstances that the varieties are not included in national level or ministerial level standard for prepared slices, the local standards of prepared slices could be used, and at the same time, they should be put on file to the Pharmaceutical supervisory and Administrative Department of the State Council. The local standards of prepared slices include *Jiangxi Provincial Specifications of PHCM*, *Fujian Provincial Specifications of PHCM*, etc.

参考文献：

[1] 王琦，孙立立，贾天柱.中药饮片炮制发展回眸[J].中成药，2000（01）：35-60.

[2] 叶喜德，徐伟，祝婧，等.中药炮制学科在中医药研究生教育发展的研究[J].江西中医药大学学报，2020，32（01）：93-96.

[3] 张志国，杨磊，张琴，等.中药炮制的现状及出现的新问题[J].中华中医药杂志，2018，33（08）：3233-3238.

[4] 石生军.浅谈中药炮制发展的现状[J].世界最新医学信息文摘，2016，16（53）：175-176.

[5] 孙娥，徐凤娟，张振海，等.中药炮制机制研究进展及研究思路探讨[J].中国中药杂志，2014，39（03）：363-369.

[6] 高飞，傅超美，胡慧玲，等.关于中药炮制机制研究现状与发展趋势的思考[J].中国实验方剂学杂志，2013，19（05）：352-355.

[7] 黄林如.中药加工炮制与临床疗效关系探究[J].中国医药科学，2012，2（18）：98+100.

[8] 张海燕.关于中药饮片的炮制[J].内蒙古中医药，2010，29（13）：103.

[9] 肖永庆，张村，李丽.中药炮制研究回顾与展望[J].世界科学技术（中医药现代化），2009，11（04）：536-540.

[10] 乔喜芹.浅析中药炮制学的基本任务[J].黑龙江医药，2007（01）：51.

Part II 第二部分

Traditional Processing of Chinese Herbal Medicine 传统炮制

第一章 传统炮制流派发展概况

中药炮制技术流派历史悠久、内容丰富、具有鲜明的地方特色。由于全国各地的药材资源、用药习惯、文化传统等多方面的差异,使不同地区的炮制技术各具特色,同时各地的大批中医师和药工,也在中药材加工炮制方面荟萃了各自的独特技艺,形成了不同的炮制技术流派。全国主要的中药炮制技术流派,根据区域位置的不同大致可以归纳为:江西的樟帮、建昌帮,四川的川帮和北京的京帮等,现将上述传统流派的发展简要概述如下。

一、樟帮的起源和发展

樟帮发源于我国江西省樟树市,为全国中药炮制的主要流派,距今有 1800 多年的历史,其炮制加工自成体系,在国内外享有较高的声誉。因此,有"药不过樟树不灵"之说。

公元 233 年(东吴嘉禾二年)至公元 244 年,葛玄(公元 164—244 年)在樟树东南的阁皂山炼丹 11 年。在炼丹的水土选择、药物药性疗效识别、鉴定、加工炮制等方面积累了丰富的经验,是樟树中药材加工炮制的创始人。唐代大批学者慕名来阁皂山学道炼丹、学医、采药行医,或兼营"药圃"。

宋代樟树医药取得了很大的发展,州府均设有官办药局,出售各种成药,私人经营的药铺不断增加,经樟树运转的药材日益频繁,樟树药业贸易进一步发展。南宋时期樟树镇已经形成"药市"。

Part II Traditional Processing of Chinese Herbal Medicine

Chapter One Summary of the Development of Traditional Schools of PCHM

PCHM technology has a long history, rich content, and distinctive local characteristics. Due to the differences in medicinal materials, medication habits, cultural traditions, and other aspects across the country, the processing technology in different regions has its characteristics. At the same time, a large number of Chinese medicine practitioners and medical workers gathered in various places and gathered their unique skills in processing, forming different processing technology schools. The main schools of TCM processing technology in China can be roughly summarized as Zhang Society in Jiangxi province, Jianchang in Jiangxi province, Chuan Society in Sichuan province, and Jing Society in Beijing. The development of the above-mentioned traditional schools is briefly summarized as follows.

Section One The Origin and Development of Zhang Society

Zhang Society originated in Zhangshu city in Jiangxi province in China. It is the main school of TCM processing with a history of more than 1800 years. Its processing system has a high reputation both at home and abroad. Therefore, there is a saying that " The medicine would not be the best effect if it's not coming from Zhangshu".

From A.D. 233 (the second year of Jiahe, Easten Wu) to A.D. 244, GeXuan (A.D.164-244) made elixir on Gezao Mountain, southeast of Zhangshu city for 11 years. He had accumulated rich experience in the selection of water and soil in alchemy, as well as the identification of medicinal properties and medicinal effect, identification, and processing. He was the founder of PCHM in Zhangshu. In the Tang Dynasty, a large number of scholars came to Gezao Mountain to learn Taoism and alchemy, to study medicine, collect herbs and practice TCM, or to run a "Chinese medicine garden" concurrently.

The medication of Zhangshu made great progress in the Song Dynasty. The state government set up a government-run medicinal affair, selling a variety of Chinese patent medicines. Private drug shops continued to increase. The medicinal materials operated by Zhangshu became more frequent, and the trade in Zhangshu pharmaceutical industry was further developed. During the Southern Song Dynasty, Zhangshu Town had formed a "drug market".

明代樟树药业空前兴盛，樟树镇有"药码头"之称。由于樟树药材品种齐全、炮制精良，樟树药材贸易范围逐渐扩大到长江、珠江流域，成为南方药材集散中心，这是形成"药不到樟树不齐"的重要因素之一。

清代初期，樟树药市出现空前兴旺，随着药业竞争的出现，全国各地药商渐渐形成帮派。樟树药商也结合成帮，即"樟帮"，并且以人数众多、经营独特、管理严密著称。樟树药工在长期的继承和实践中，总结整理古人中药炮制经验及各派成就，将药物性能与临床紧密结合，开创了"樟帮"独特的炮制风格。

2013年，樟树被中国中药协会授予"中国药都"荣誉称号。

二、建昌帮的起源和发展

建昌药业的起源，得益于东晋时期医药学家葛洪和唐代一些道教人士在南城县（古称建昌府）的医药活动。因此，建昌药业的起源至少可追溯到晋代。

宋代袁燮为建昌撰写的《建昌军药局记》载有"若古先民，念斯民受病之苦也，非药不去。而药之为性，有温、有热、有寒、有平，其品不一，于是乎名之曰君、曰臣、曰使、曰佐，而为制之方，精切微密，毫发不差，随其病而施之。而罔市利者，辄欲以琐琐私意而增损剂量之可乎……若夫较计纤悉，急于牟利，药不及精，与市肆所鬻无别"。说明到宋代时建昌人已讲求药物质量和药效精良，能够改变药性、制备药物，可有目的性地使用药物以适应临床治疗的需要。因此，从宋代时起讲求药物质量和药业信誉便已成为建昌药业发展的方向。

In the Ming Dynasty, the medicine industry of Zhangshu was unprecedentedly prosperous, and Yushu Town was known as the "Yao Matou (dock of medicine)". Due to the complete variety and excellent processing of medicinal materials in Zhangshu, the scope of the trade of medicinal materials in Zhangshu has gradually expanded to the Yangtze River and Pearl River basins, becoming the distribution center of southern medicinal materials. This was one of the important factors for the formation of "In Zhangshu there has the most complete range of medicines".

In the early Qing Dynasty, the drug market of Zhangshu flourished unprecedentedly. With the emergence of competition in the medicine company, the competition was becoming more and more fierce, the medical schools were formed gradually. There was a unique school in Zhangshu, which was called "Zhang Society". "Zhang Society" was famous for its large number, unique processing operation, and strict management. In the long-term inheritance and practice, pharmaceutical workers in Zhangshu summarized and sorted out the processing experiences and achievements of different schools from ancients times, closely combining the medicinal properties with clinical practice, and created the unique processing style of "Zhang Society".

Zhangshu was awarded the honorary title of "Chinese Medicine Capital" by the China Association of Traditional Chinese Medicine in 2013.

Section Two   The Origin and Development of Jianchang Society

The origin of the Jianchang medicine industry was due to the medical activities of Ge Hong, a medical expert in the Eastern Jin Dynasty, and some Taoists in the Tang Dynasty in Nancheng County (called "Jianchang Prefecture" in ancient time). Therefore, the origin of the Jianchang medicine industry can be traced back at least to the Jin Dynasty.

The *Records of Jianchang Military Medicine Bureau* written by Yuan Xie in the Song Dynasty for Jianchang contain the following words: "If the ancient people think of sufferings of diseases, they chose medicine to treat with. And the medicinal properties include warm, hot, cold, and neutral, its medicinal properties are different, and just like the monarch, minister, assistant, and guide, while the dispensing prescriptions have accurate dosage, and it should be prescribed the medicine according to the symptoms. Those who value interests always try their best to increase or decrease dosage to get the best benefit. If you are calculating and eager to make profits, not caring about the best use of the drugs, it is no different from normal shop-bought and sold." These sentences show that in Song Dynasty, the Jianchang people had emphasized the quality and efficacy of medicines, and could change the nature of medicines, and purposefully use medicines to meet the needs of clinical treatment. Therefore, from Song Dynasty, it had become the director of the development of the Jianchang medicine Industry to emphasize the reliability of the quality and reputation of medicines.

著名的医类方书《瑞竹堂经验方》为我国古代医药学史上一部有较高价值的著作，反映了元代建昌药业的用药、制药状况。该书收载了炒、炮、煨、煅、炙、水飞等药材加工炮制方法，各药的制备要求也非常严格。从《瑞竹堂经验方》的内容可看到元代建昌人对药物的认识和应用已达很高水平，不仅能够制备出各种药物剂型，并且每一味药的加工炮制和使用方法都非常细致规范。《瑞竹堂经验方》不仅是元代建昌人对前人用药经验的总结，对后代建昌医药也有深远的影响。

明清时期是建昌药业发展鼎盛的时期。建昌药业在明代、清代几百年间经历了质的升华，在饮片加工炮制和经营销售方面形成特色，并在相当长的时期保持着繁荣昌盛的状态，建昌药业便自然而然地在此期间形成药帮——建昌帮，在药界赢得了信誉和地位。

三、川帮的起源和发展

四川素有"中医之乡""中药之库"之称，早在唐宋时期，四川就有49种道地药材，为全国之最。尤其是成都地区，由于悠久的历史文化和深厚浓郁的中医药文化相结合，使成都成为全国著名的中医药之乡，有一大批知名的中医师和药工云集在这座历史文化名城，并逐渐形成了独具风格的地方中药炮制特色，称为"川帮"，并与江西的"樟帮""建昌帮"，京津地区的"京帮"并称为中药炮制技艺的四大帮。

在20世纪50年代以前，成都尚有大小药房近百家，基本上都采用"前店后坊"的经营模式，从事中医治病和药材炮制。川帮的中药炮制技术具有良好的传统和基础，但是由于中医传承的固有规律，如药物炮制的火候大多是靠师徒间的口传心授，其经验性、主观判断性的因素较强。因此，随着实践经验丰富的老药工逐渐谢世，一批中药炮制技术也面临着消亡或变异的危险，亟须进一步继承和发扬。

At the same time, the famous medical prescription book *Ruizhutang Experience Prescription* is a valuable work in the history of ancient Chinese medicine, which reflects the medication and pharmaceutical status of the Jianchang Pharmaceutical Industry in the Yuan Dynasty. The book contains the processing methods of stir-frying, baking, roasting, calcination, stir-frying with liquid assistants, grinding with water, and other processing technologies and the processing requirements are also very strict. The content of *Ruizhutang Experience Prescription* showed that in the Yuan Dynasty, Jianchang people had a high level of understanding to know how to use the medicine. They could not only prepare various medicines dosage forms but also process each medicine with precise and standard methods. *Ruizhutang Experience Prescription* is not only a summary of the experience of processing technologies by Jianchang people in the Yuan Dynasty but also has a far-reaching impact on Jianchang medicine for future generations.

The period of the Ming and Qing Dynasties was the period of prosperous development of the Jianchang medicine industry. Jianchang medicine industry experienced a process of qualitative sublimation and development during the centuries of Ming and Qing Dynasties. It formed its characteristics in processing and marketing and maintained a prosperous state for quite a long time. From then on, Jianchang medicine industry naturally formed a medicine school, called Jianchang Society, which had won the reputation and status in the Chinese medicine industry.

Section Three   The Origin and Development of Chuan Society

Sichuan is known as "the hometown of traditional Chinese medicine, the storehouse of traditional Chinese herbal medicine". As early as the Tang and Song Dynasties, there were 49 authentic medicinal materials in Sichuan province, which was the largest amount in the country. Especially in the Chengdu area, due to the combination of long history culture and strong traditional Chinese medicine culture, Chengdu had become a famous hometown of traditional Chinese medicine in China. A large number of well-known Chinese physicians and pharmacists gathered in this historic and cultural city, and gradually formed a unique style with local traditional Chinese medicine processing characteristics, known as "Chuan Society", and with the "Zhang Society", "Jianchang Society" in Jiangxi, and the "Jing Society" in Beijing and Tianjin, they are all known as the four major Societies in the processing technology of traditional Chinese medicine.

Before the 1950s, there were nearly 100 Chinese medicine pharmacies in Chengdu, which adopted the business model of "front shop and back workshop", engaged in traditional Chinese medicine treatment and processing of medicinal materials. The processing technology of traditional Chinese medicine in Chuan Society has a good tradition and foundation. However, due to the limitation of the traditional TCM inherent law, for example, imparting processing skills only through oral teaching between teachers and apprentices, with strong empiric and subjectivity. As the gradually passed away of experienced veteran pharmacists, some unique traditional processing technologies also in danger of extinction or variation, which urgently needs further inheritance and development.

四、京帮的起源和发展

京帮炮制技术流派发源于我国北京,其代表饮片包括"九转胆星"和"酒蒸大黄"等。京帮发展至今,其炮制的特点主要体现在炮制方法和辅料特色上。

清代有京帮的说法,但当时并未强调这一称谓,而是称为京通卫帮,也就是涵盖了北京、通州、天津卫,当时也有分别称为京帮、通州帮、天津卫帮等。沿用至今,统称为京帮,但仍涵盖了三个地区。

Section Four The Origin and Development of Jing Society

Jing Society processing technology originated in Beijing, China, its representative decoction pieces including "Jiuzhuan Bile Arisaema" and "Steamed Rhei Radix Et Rhizoma with Wine" and so on.

In the Qing Dynasty, there has been saying about Jiang Society but without emphasizing, sometimes also called Jingtongwei Society, which includes the processing technologies from the districts of Beijing, Tongzhou, and Tianjingwei, sometimes they are separately called Jing Society, Tongzhou Society, and Tianjingwei Society, till now, Jing Society becomes a formal name, containing processing technologies from these three districts.

参考文献：

[1]周建芽，龚千锋."樟帮"中医药文化的精神特质及发展展望[J].江西中医药大学学报，2017，29（04）：103-105.

[2]钟凌云，于欢，祝婧，等.炮制技术流派——樟树帮药文化探究[J].中国实验方剂学杂志，2017，23（02）：1-6.

[3]钟凌云，龚千锋，杨明，等.传统炮制技术流派特点及发展[J].中国中药杂志，2013，38（19）：3405-3408.

[4]龚千锋，祝婧，周道根.樟树药帮的历史与特色[J].江西中医学院学报，2007（04）：27-28.

[5]郭三保，何芹，周铁文，等.建昌帮发展历程及炮制特色探究[J].中国中医药现代远程教育，2021，19（06）：80-82.

[6]徐春娟，陈荣，何晓晖.旴江医著《瑞竹堂经验方》探析[J].中国实验方剂学杂志，2016，22（18）：183-186.

[7]钟凌云，龚千锋，杨明.建昌帮炮制技术传承与发展初探[J].江西中医药，2015，46（09）：7-10

[8] 吴蜀瑶，李洋，吴志瑰，等.建昌药帮的传统炮制特色［J］.江西中医药，2016，47（11）：11-14.

[9] 杨冰，蔡宝昌，张洪雷.江西省中药文化软实力［J］.江西科学，2017，35（02）：318-322.

[10] 颜冬梅，李娜，张金莲，等.江西传统炮制技术的研究进展［J］.中药材，2016，39（02）：447-450.

[11] 李梦琪，罗林，尚宁宁，等.从文化传承到产业现代化的矛盾与对策探究中药炮制现状［J］.中成药，2020，42（11）：2999-3003.

[12] 杨殿兴，田兴军.川派中医药源流与发展［M］.北京：中国中医药出版社，2016.

[13] 洪巧瑜，卜训生，李飞，等.以京帮流派中药炮制方法为指导的中药炮制继承教学体系探讨［J］.中国医药导报，2019，16（13）：120-123+131.

［14］杨明，钟凌云，薛晓，等.中药传统炮制技术传承与创新［J］.中国中药杂志，2016，41（03）：357-361.

［15］隋丞琳，顾选，朱力，等.浅析京帮炮制技术传承与发展［J］.北京中医药，2018，37（04）：363-365.

［16］王炯，杨小源.王子义京帮流派中药炮制制备工艺探析［J］.西部中医药，2013，26（07）：31-33.

［17］顾选，刘青，隋丞琳，等.北京地区传统中药饮片特色品种初探［J］.中药材，2018，41（03）：581-584.

［18］李莉，姚峥嵘，王艳翚.中药老字号配方及炮制技术保护现状及思考［J］.中国药房，2018，29（09）：1171-1175.

第二章 各流派的炮制特点

一、樟帮的炮制特点

樟帮的中药炮制技术，不论炒、炙、浸、泡或烘、晒、藏均十分考究，独树一帜，炮制工具、辅料和工艺均具有鲜明的地方特色。

1. 加工炮制工具

樟帮中药炮制技艺在不断总结完善的过程中，创造了一套自己独特的传统加工炮制工具。主要有：铡刀、片刀、刮刀、铁锚、碾槽、冲钵、蟹钳、鹿茸加工壶、压板和硫黄药柜等。尤其是片刀、铡刀面小口薄，轻便锋利，被称为"樟刀"，有着"老君炉中纯火青，炼就樟刀叶片轻，锋利好比鸳鸯剑，飞动如飞饮片精"的美誉。

2. 饮片炮制工艺

（1）切制工艺：樟帮的中药炮制，提倡制虽繁、不惜工，一丝不苟，其精湛工艺切制的中药饮片以薄如纸、吹得起、断面齐、造型美而久负盛名。饮片工艺独具风格，如可将1寸长的白芍切成360片等，有"白芍飞上天，木通不见边，陈皮一条线，半夏鱼鳞片，肉桂薄肚片，黄柏骨牌片，甘草柳叶片，桂枝瓜子片，枳壳凤眼片，川芎蝴蝶双飞片，一粒马钱子切206片（腰子片），槟榔切108片"的切制方法和工艺，被誉为"鬼斧神工，不类凡品"。

Chapter Two Processing Characteristics of Different Schools of PCHM

Section One Processing Technology Characteristics of Zhang Society

The processing technology in Zhang Society, whether frying, stir-frying with liquid, dipping, soaking or baking, sun-drying or storing, are all very sophisticated and unique, with distinct local characteristics in processing tools, processing assistants, and procedure.

1. Processing tools

In the progress of continuous improvement and perfection of TCM processing technology in Zhang Society, a unique set of traditional processing tools were created. It mainly includes: sickle, slicing knife, scraper, iron anchor, grinding trough, punching, crab claws, antler processing pot, pressure plate, and sulfur medicine cabinet. In particular, the slicing knife and sickle are unnormal. The surfaces of the slicing knife and sickle are small and thin, light and sharp, being called "Zhang knives". It has a famous reputation, and there's a poem to prove it: "the pure fire in the Laojun's furnace refines the light of the blade of the Zhang knife, the sharpness of the knife is better than that of the sword, and the flying of the knife is like the flying decoction piece".

2. Processing technology of decoction pieces

(1) Cutting process: In Zhang Society processing, it is advocates that although the processing is complicated, the labor should strive for perfection with scrupulous care. The traditional Chinese medicine decoction pieces cut with their exquisite craftsmanship have long been famous for being as thin as paper, able to be blown, with a clean section and beautiful shape. The cutting technology is unique, for example, the one-inch-long Paeoniae Radix Alba (Baishao) could be cut into 360 pieces, etc. There are sayings of "Paeoniae Radix Alba (Baishao) pieces could fly into the sky for the light and thin; Akebiae Caulis (Mutong) pieces should be very thin without obvious rim, Citri Reticulatae Pericarpium (Chenpi) pieces show as a line, Corydalis Rhizoma (Banxia) is cut into pieces like fish scales, Cinnamon Cortex (Rougui) are cut into pieces like thin tripe, Phellodendri Chinensis Cortex (Huangbai) are cut into pieces like dominoes, Glycyrrhizae Radix Et Rhizoma (Gancao) pieces show as willow leaves, Cinnamomi Ramulus (Guizhi) pieces show as melon seeds, Aurantii Fructus (Zhike) pieces like double phoenix eyes, Chuanxiong Rhizoma (chuanxiong) pieces like butterfly flying, one Strychni Semen (Maqianzi) could be cut into 206 pieces (reniform like pieces) and Arecae Semen (Binglang) could be cut into 108 pieces ". These pieces are known as "The skillful workmanship that it's unusual".

此外，在李时珍的《本草纲目》和现代的《中药大辞典》中均有记载的中洲枳壳，在切制前还要经过特殊的发酵工艺处理，发酵后切制的饮片皮青、肉厚、色白、香味浓、果囊小，呈凤眼状，被称为"枳壳凤眼片"，为枳壳中之上品。

（2）炒制法：樟帮的炒制法包括了微炒、小火炒、炒黄和炒爆四大类。

①微炒：不直接在锅内炒，以防止药物焦化或灰化而降低药效。如炒葶苈子，取净原药置垫纸的锅内炒（在纸上炒），炒至纸焦黄为度，樟帮又称之为"纸上炒"。其炒制目的是炒后性缓，适宜患病夹虚者。

②小火炒：用较小的火，将药物炒热、炒香，其颜色性味不变，樟帮称"去味去臭，色性不变"。其目的是矫味、矫臭，清除药物表面的霉菌等。如炒五谷虫，即用小火炒至五谷虫外表约焦黄色、发香为度，略透明，质松脆易碎，断面多空泡，至无臭味。其炒制目的是炒后焦香入脾，增强健脾、消疳积的作用。

③炒黄：炒至表面微黄色鼓起，以能嗅到药物散发固有的气味为度。樟帮称"黄而不焦，香气四溢"。如炒牵牛子，即用小火炒至鼓起、发响、表面淡黄色（白牵牛子）、有香气为度。

④炒爆：多用于种子类药物，加热炒使种子爆裂、香气透出，除去闷人气味，使体积膨胀，易于成分煎出。樟帮称"逢子必炒，药香溢街"。

In addition, the Zhongzhou Aurantii Fructus (Zhike), which is recorded in Li Shizhen's *Compendium of Materia Medica* and *The Dictionary of Medicinal Plant*, has to undergo a special fermentation process before being cut. After fermentation, the pieces have green skin, with thick pericarp, white color, strong fragrance, and small fruit sac, showing phoenix-eyes shape, being called "Fructus Aurantii Pieces as phoenix eye", which is the top quality products in Aurantii Fructus (Zhike) pieces.

(2) Stir-frying method: The stir-frying methods of Zhang Society include stir-frying on paper, stir-frying with little heat, stir-frying with low heat, and crack-frying:

① **Stir-frying on paper:** Don't stir-fry directly in the pot to prevent coking or ashing of drugs to avoid the reduce the efficacy. For example, stir-frying Descurainiae Semen Lepidii Semen (Tinglizi), place the original drug in a paper-padded pot (stir-fry on paper), stir-fry until the paper becomes brown, also called "Stir-frying on paper". The purpose of this method is to moderate the medicinal properties and make it suit for weak patients.

② **Stir-frying with little heat:** To stir-fry drugs with little heat, the color and taste of drugs remain unchanged, called "Deodorizing and deodorizing, and the color is unchanged" in Zhang Society. The purpose is to correct taste and odor and remove the mold on the surface of the drug. For example, stir-frying grain worms, using little heat to fry until the appearance of the worms shows burnt yellow slightly transparent and smells burnt, the texture becomes crisp and brittle, the cross-section shows more vacuoles and with no odor. The purpose of this frying is to make drugs burnt and easy to affect the spleen channel, enhance the effect of invigorating the spleen, and eliminating malnutrition.

③ **stir-frying with low heat:** Stir-fry drugs with low heat until the appearance shows yellowish, expansion, as well as smell the inherent odor of the drugs. Also called "yellow without burning, fragrance overflowing" in Zhang Society. For example, stir-frying Pharbitidis Semen (Qianniuzi) with low heat until it is expansion, the poping sound could be heard and the appearance of the drug shows yellow with aroma smell.

④ **Crack-frying:** This method is mostly suited for seed drugs. Crack-frying would make seeds burst and the fragrance permeate, the stuffy odor removed and show expansion, the effective components in the drug would be easy to decoct out. There's a saying about this, "Stir-fry every seed to make drug fragrance overflowing the street" in Zhang Society.

（3）辅料制法：樟帮对辅料非常讲究，既有"樟树中药炮制，辅料讲究地道，归经如择，用量适度，疗效增强"的说法，又有"术遵岐伯，法效雷公"之训。例如，酒用糯米酒、醋用新年米醋、蜜用橙花蜜、米用糙米、土用灶心土或陈壁土，并且要求炮制须考虑辅料归经和用量。辅料包括固体辅料和液体辅料，其中固体辅料有油砂、蛤粉、滑石粉、糙米、灶心土、麦麸、白矾等；液体辅料有酒、醋、盐水、姜水、蜜汁、甘草汁、皂角汁、乳汁、米泔水、山羊血、猪心血、鳖血、胆汁、羊脂油、童便等。

樟帮比较独特的辅料制法和品种包括：

①猪心血炒酸枣仁：取新鲜猪心，剖开挤出血，用清水适量稀释，再与酸枣仁拌润，待吸尽，置铜锅内，用小火炒至干为度。猪心血有宁心、敛汗、生津的功效，猪心血炒酸枣仁可增强宁心安神的作用，对虚烦不眠、惊悸多梦有奇特的疗效。

②甘草汁、皂角汁制草乌：以甘草汁、皂角汁炮制草乌，降低其毒性。

③童便制马钱子：樟树用童便制马钱子已有一千多年的历史。经实验研究，童便制马钱子含士的宁0.389%，而生马钱子含士的宁1.905%，可有效降低马钱子毒性成分含量。

④鳖血炒柴胡：取柴胡片，用鳖血加温水稀释拌匀，稍闷润至吸干水分为度，置铜锅内，用小火炒至药物表面呈黄褐色。其目的是抑制升浮之性，增强清肝退热之功。对因疟疾类引起的肝脾肿大，效果奇佳，截疟功效显著。

第二部分 传统炮制
Part II Traditional Processing of Chinese Herbal Medicine

(3) Processing with assistant materials: Assistant materials in processing in Zhang Society are very important. It has said that "Assistant materials in processing in Zhang Society are very authentic, the channel tropism should be chosen, dosage should be moderate and curative effect should be enhanced", there is also a saying that "following the medical skills of Qi Bo (famous ancient Chinese physician) and processing methods of Lei Xiao (famous ancient Chinese pharmacist)". For example, the assistant material of wine should be glutinous rice wine, the assistant material of vinegar should be rice vinegar, the assistant material of honey should be orange nectar honey, the assistant material of rice should be brown rice, the assistant material of soil should be stove subsoil or soil on an ancient wall. Except that, the channels affected by processing assistant materials and the dosages should be carefully considered before the assistant materials used in processing. The assistant materials include solid and liquid styles. For the solid assistant materials, oil sands, clam meal, talcum powder, brown rice, stove subsoil, wheat bran, alum, and so on are included. For the liquid assistant materials, liquor, vinegar, saltwater, ginger juice, honey juice, Glycyrrhizae Radix Et Rhizoma juice, Gleditsia Sinensis Fructus juice, milk, rice bran water, goat blood, pig heart blood, soft-shelled turtle blood, bile, mutton fat oil, urine of boys and so on are included. The unique processing methods and varieties of assistant materials in Zhang Society include:

① **Stir frying Ziziphi Spinosae Semen (Suanzaoren) with pig's heart's blood:** Take fresh pig heart, slitting and squeeze bleeding, dilute it with clear water, and then mix it with Ziziphi Spinosae Semen (Suanzaoren). After the blood is absorbed by the drug, put them together in a copper pot, stir-fry it with low heat until it is dry. The pig's heart's blood has the effect of calming the mind and arresting sweating and generating body fluids. Stir-frying Ziziphi Spinosae Semen (Suanzaoren) with pig's heart's blood can enhance the function of relieving mental stress and calm the mind. It has peculiar curative effects on insomnia, palpitation, and dreaminess.

② **Glycyrrhizae Radix Et Rhizoma juice preparation and saponin juice preparation:** Aconiti Kusnezoffii Radix (Caowu) could be processed with Glycyrrhizae Radix Et Rhizoma juice and saponin horn juice to reduce its toxicity.

③ **Boy's urine processed Strychni Semen (Maqianzi):** This method of processing Strychni Semen (Maqianzi) with boy's urine in Zhangshu has been used for more than a thousand years. The experimental results showed that the contents of strychnine were 0.389%, and 1.905% in Strychni Semen (Maqianzi) processed with boy's urine strychnine and in raw Strychni Semen separately, which means the method could effectively reduce the toxic components of Strychni Semen (Maqianzi).

④ **Stir-frying Bupleuri Radix (Chaihu) with soft-shelled turtle blood:** mix Bupleuri Radix (Chaihu) slices with soft-shelled turtle blood diluted by warm water, moisten in a short time until the blood is absorbed. Place them together in a copper pot and stir-fry them with low heat until the surface of the drug shows brown. The purpose is to inhibit the drug's rise and fall properties, enhance the function of clearing the liver, and reducing fever. For the disease of liver and spleen enlargement caused by malaria, the effect is excellent and the effect of malaria control is remarkable.

另外，还有油砂炒（鳖甲）、蛤粉炒（阿胶）、滑石粉炒（黄狗肾）、糙米炒（斑蝥）、灶心土或陈壁土炒（白术）、麦麸炒（枳壳）、酒炒（当归）、醋炒（青皮）、盐水炒（杜仲）、姜汁炒（厚朴）、山羊血制（藤黄）、羊脂油炒（淫羊藿）、豆腐制（藤黄）、明矾制（白附子）、米泔水制（白术）、蜜炙（甘草）等，独特的辅料炮制方法和品种成为樟帮中药炮制技术流派的主要特色之一。

二、建昌帮的炮制特点

建昌传统中药炮制方法是历代从事医药行业的人们不断积累和发展起来的。建昌帮以中药饮片加工炮制和集散经营销售两方面特色著称。在饮片炮制方面，最著名的就是炮制工具、辅料和工艺独具传统风格，讲求形、色、气、味俱全，毒性低，疗效高。

1. 加工炮制工具

建昌帮炮制工具，在刀具、刨具、筛具及辅助工具等方面具有独特性，可归纳为：刀刨齐全，特色工具多。

（1）刀具：与樟帮的樟刀相比，建昌帮的切药刀"建刀"刀把长、面大、线直、刃深，并且吃硬和省力，还可一刀多用，由建刀切制的特色饮片，往往斜、薄、大、光，外形精美而实用，如有延胡索鱼鳞片、赤芍竹叶片、防风飞上天等。

豚刀（建刀）是建昌帮最具特色的加工工具，是全国有名的三种中药加工刀之一（另两种是禹州大圆型禹刀、樟帮小刀面汉刀）。药界有"见刀认帮""刀法不同，建刀更有用"的说法。

In addition, there are other methods processed by different assistant materials, such as stir-frying with oil sand (Trionycis Carapax-Biejia), stir-frying with clam meal (Asini Corii Colla-Ejiao), stir-frying with talcum powder (Dog penis-Huanggoushen), stir-frying with brown rice (Mylabris-Banmao), stir-frying with stove subsoil or soil on ancient wall (Atractylodis Macrocephalae Rhizoma-Baizhu), stir-frying with wheat bran (Aurantii Fructus-Zhike), stir-frying with wine (Angelicae Sinensis Radix-Danggui), stir-frying with vinegar (Citri Reticulatae Pericarpium Viride-Qinpi), stir-frying with salted water (Eucommiae Cortex-Duzhong), stir-frying with ginger juice (Magnoliae Officinalis Cortex-Houpu), stir-frying with goat blood (Gamboge-Tenghuang), stir-frying with mutton fat oil (Epimedii Folium-Yinyanghuo), processing with tofu (Gamboge-Tenghuang), processing with alum (Typhonii Rhizoma-Baifuzi), processing with water from washing rice (Atractylodis Macrocephalae Rhizoma-Baizhu), stir-frying with honey (Glycyrrhizae Radix Et Rhizoma-Gancao), etc. The unique processing methods and varieties of assistant materials have become one of the main characteristics of the processing technology of Zhang Society.

Section Two Processing Technology Characteristics of Jianchang Society

The processing method of traditional Chinese medicine in Jianchang is accumulated and developed by the people who engaged in the medical industry in past dynasties. Jianchang Society is famous for its two characteristics: PCHM and the distribution and sales of drugs. For PCHM in Jiangchang Society, the best aspects are unique processing tools, assistant materials, and technologies, the medical slices or pieces are all with the best shape, color, smell, and taste, with low toxicity and high efficacy.

1. Processing Tools

Jianchang Society processing tools, including unique cutters, planers, screening tools, and auxiliary tools. These tools have a complete range of kinds with special styles.

(1) Cutter: Compared with the cutting knife in Zhang Society, the Cutters in Jianchang Society has a longer handle, a larger surface with a straight line and deep blade, it's hard and labor-saving. It can also be used as a multi-purpose knife. The shape of the special pieces cut by the tools in Jianchang Society is often oblique, thin, large, and bright, with exquisite and practical appearance, such as the fish-scale like shape slices of Corydalis Rhizoma (Yanhusuo), bamboo leaves like shape slices of Paeoniae Radix Rubra (Chi Shao), and the thin slices of Saposhnikoviae Radix (Fangfeng) which could fly into the sky for the thin and light, etc.

Dolphin-like knife (Jian Dao) is the most distinctive processing tool in Jianchang Society. It is one of the three famous Chinese medicine processing knives throughout the country (the other two are large round Yu knives in Yuzhou and small knives "Mian Han knife" in Zhang Society). There is a saying in the pharmaceutical industry that "seeing the knife and you can recognize which Society it belongs to ", "Cutting method is different, but with Jianchang Society's knife is better".

（2）雷公刨：是由建昌帮创制的独特刨具，相传发明已久并沿用至今，以操作时声大如雷而得名。以雷公刨加工饮片，不仅可使饮片薄而效力高，并且刨出药片以纵片为多，均匀美观。

（3）筛具：如泽门笼、附子筛等针对专门药物设计的筛药工具，体现了建昌帮饮片精加工的特点。

（4）其他辅助工具：多以铜、铁、木、陶等各种材质制作而成，如木制枳壳榨，用于枳壳的成型制作；铁制槟榔榉，用于槟榔的拿取切制；还有用于捣碎香附的香附铲、切制茯苓的茯苓刀、贮藏用的药坛、蒸制饮片用的圆木甑、用于磨刀的猪肝色刀石，还有麦芽篓等，都各具特色。

2. 炮制辅料

在辅料方面，建昌帮有选料独特、遵古道地、制备考究、一物多用的特点。其中尤以谷糠炒最有特色，如有谷糠煨、煅制药材，蜜糠炒炙多种药材，同时谷糠还用于净选、润制、吸湿、密封养护等。在现行主流的炮制辅料中，麦麸是用于炒制药物的重要介质，但在建昌帮的炮制技术中，少见麦的应用，而多以谷糠替代，使"南糠北麸"成为南北药帮炮制流派的一个显著区别。

除此之外，在净选、润制、吸湿、密封养护等炮制过程中，谷糠的充分应用，也体现了谷糠一物多用的特点。另外，白矾、朴硝、童便、米泔水、硫黄、砂子等，也都运用在各种建昌帮炮制中，体现其选料独特之处。

(2) Leigong planer: It is a unique planer that originated from Jianchang Society. It has been invented for a long time and until now it is still be used. The name of "Leigong" came from its loud sound during operation (like thundering). To get slices or pieces of Chinese Materia Medica with Leigong planer can not only make slices thin and effective but also make slices more lengthwise, uniform, and beautiful.

(3) Screening tools: This kind of tool is special for screen drugs with different sizes, such as Zemen cage and Aconiti Lateralis Radix Praeparata screen, the tools reflect the characteristics of delicate processing in Jianchang Society.

(4) Other auxiliary tools: The other auxiliary tools of processing in Jianchang Society are mostly made of various materials, such as copper, iron, or wood, for example, the wooden pottery special for processing Aurantii Fructus (Zhike), which is used for the molding of Aurantii Fructus (Zhike) to make phoenix eyes-like slices. Betel beech made of iron is used for the catch and cut of betel nut. The Cyperi Rhizoma (Xiangfu) shovel just for mashing the Cyperi Rhizoma (Xiangfu), the Poria (Fuling) knife for the preparation of Poria (Fuling), the medicine jar for storage drugs, the round wooden steamer for steaming decoction pieces, the auburn color knife stone for sharpening knives, the malt basket for processing malt, and so on. All the tools have their characteristics.

2. Processing assistant material

The characteristics of the processing assistant materials in Jianchang Society include that the selection of assistant materials, the processing methods with assistant materials are unique, authentic, and exquisite, sometimes, the assistant materials are not only used as assistants but can be used in other ways. Among these assistant materials, the rice bran is the most special assistant, which is not only used for simmering, calcining, and stir-frying drugs, but also can be used for cleaning, lubrication, moisture absorption, sealing, and maintenance. Wheat bran is an important medium for stir-frying in the current mainstream of processing assistant materials, but in the processing technology of Jianchang Society, wheat bran is rarely used and replaced by rice bran, which makes "south rice bran north wheat bran" a significant difference in the processing schools of north and south PCHM gang.

In addition, in the process of cleaning, moistening, hygroscopicity, sealing, and maintenance, the full application of rice bran also embodies the characteristics of multipurpose rice bran. In addition, alum, sodium sulfate, boy's urine, water in which rice has been washed, sulfur, sand, etc. are also used in all kinds of Jianchang Society processing, reflecting its unique selection of materials.

3. 炮制工艺

因奉行药食同源的原则，自古以来，建昌帮炮制工艺就多取法于烹饪技术，以水制、火制和水火共制作为保证建昌帮中药饮片质量的重要手段，而火制和水火共制又与烹调技术紧密关联，从而形成基于烹饪特色的建昌帮炮制技术特点。建昌帮遵循的炮制原则是"炮制虽繁，必不得省工夫；辅料虽贵，必不得短斤两"，体现出"水火不失其度，炮制精细逞其巧妙"的应用。

在水制方面，建昌帮技术强调四季水性的差异，有冬水善，夏水恶的说法，认为不明水性，就不懂水制。润制药材要看水头，即强调要善于判断药材软化的程度，总结出"久洗无药味，久泡无药气，少泡多润莫伤水，无气无味卖药渣"等水制法的传统经验。

在火制方面，建昌帮对文武火候的运用多有建树，其充分吸取了烹饪技术中武火急速快炒的特点，对建昌帮饮片的炮制也提出了类似要求，通过该方法的加工，可达到饮片色艳而气香的目的；而当用文火进行煨制处理时，又可体现饮片纯真而味厚的特点，同时减毒增效，如煨附片等。

在水火共制方面，炙制姜半夏、炆熟地黄、酒洗当归等，均为建昌帮的特色饮片。

3. Processing technology

Due to the principle of homologous medicine and food, since ancient times, the processing technology of Jianchang Society has been mostly based on cooking technology. Processing with water, fire, and water-fire co-production are important means to ensure the quality of Chinese herbal slices processed with Jianchang Society processing technologies, and processing with fire and water-fire co-production are closely related to cooking techniques, to form the characteristics of the processing technique based on the characteristics of cooking. The principle of Jianchang Society PCHM follows that processing is complex, must not save time; accessories, although expensive, must not give short weight. It reflects the request that processing with fire and water should keep suitable operation, and delicate processing is necessary for the best curative effect of Chinese herbal slices.

In terms of processing with water, The difference in water quality in four seasons is emphasized in Jianchang Society PCHM technology. There is a saying that water is good in winter and bad in summer, if you don't know about water, you don't know how to process drugs with water. Moistening medicinal materials should depend on water, that is, to be good at judging the extent of softening medicinal materials, Traditional experiences of processing with water were summed up as, long-time washing makes no medicinal taste, long-time foaming makes no medical effect, less foaming and more moistening keep drugs from lost of the medical effect, the drugs without medical effects equal to invalid dregs.

In the aspect of processing with fire, there are many experiences in Jianchang Society PCHM. The pharmacists fully absorbed the characteristics of rapid and quick fry with high heat in cooking technology and put forward similar requests in Jianchang Society PCHM. Through the processing of this method, the decoction pieces can be colorful and fragrant. And when simmering drugs with low heat, the slices or pieces show the characteristics with pure effect, at the same time the toxicity could be reduced, such as simmering Aconiti Lateralis Radix Praeparata (Fuzi).

In the aspect of processing with water-fire co-production, processed Pinelliae Rhizoma (Banxia) with ginger, prepared rhizome of rehmannia (Shudihuang) processed by braising, Angelicae Sinensis Radix (Danggui) washed by liquor are all special pieces in Jianchang Society.

在建昌帮炮制十三法（炒、炙、煨、煅、蒸、煮、炆、熬、淬、霜、作曲、发芽、复制和其他制法）中，尤以炒、炙、煨、炆、蒸法工艺特色为多，其中炆法属于建昌帮独有的传统炮制方法。"炆"原指没有火焰的微火，方言中指用微火炖食物或熬菜。建昌帮炆法炮制工艺为：取净药材，加水浸透后，放入炆药罐内，加入清水，上盖，移至围灶内，罐周围堆满干糠，点火炆2～3天，中途加入辅料拌匀，炆至糠尽灰冷，药熟汁干时取出，干燥。《江西省中药饮片炮制规范（2008年版）》共收载4种炆法炮制品，炆地黄、炆何首乌、炆黄精、炆远志。

《建昌帮传统中药炮制法》（梅开丰等著）对建昌帮中药炮制特色和100多味中药的建昌传统炮制工艺方法也作了详细的叙述。

三、川帮的炮制特点

川帮的中医药发展具有悠久的历史。川帮发源于我国四川省，以庚鼎药房、精益堂为代表，以"九制大黄""九转南星""仙半夏"等特色炮制品种闻名，其中，比较著名的川产临江片（或称熟片）流传有较详细的炮制方法，即洗泥后，用胆水加清水混合，将附子放入浸泡后，放到锅内煮至过心，浸泡、剥皮、再用清水浸，然后横切成厚片，再以浸泡至转色面后入蒸笼蒸透，火力须掌握均匀，不能中途停火，如此蒸出来的附片质量良好，有油面，有光泽，蒸好后放在烤席上用木炭火烤，火力勿过大，烘干后即成熟片。

Among the thirteen methods in Jianchang Society PCHM (stir-frying, roasting, simmering, calcining, steaming, boiling, braising, stewing, quenching, frosting, ferment, sprouting, complex process, and other methods), the processing methods of stir-frying, roasting, simmering, braising and steaming are with more characteristic, especially the method of braising which is the unique processing technology in Jianchang Society. "braising" originally refers to light fire without flame. In dialect, it refers to stewing food or boiling vegetables with light fire. The braising processing technology in Jianchang Society is as follows: take the pure medicinal materials, soak them with water, put them into the pot, add water, cover the pot, move them to the kitchen range, pile up the dry rice bran around the pot, ignite and heat for 2-3 days, mix some assistant materials during processing, keep heating until the rice bran becomes ashy and cold, the juice in the pot is absorbed by drugs completely, take out the drugs and make them dry. There are four products processed by braising technology record in *Jiangxi Provincial rules for PCHM* (edition in 2008), including braised Rehmanniae Radix (Dihuang), braised Polygonum Multiflorum Radix (Heshouwu), braised Polygonati Rhizoma (Huangjing), braised Polygalae Radix root (Yuanzhi).

Jianchang Society Traditional Chinese Herbal Processing Methods (Compiled by Mei Kaifeng et al.) described in detail the characteristics of processing technologies and more than 100 kinds of PCHM methods in Jianchang Society.

Section Three　　Processing Technology Characteristics of Chuan Society

The Chuan Society PCHM has a long history, originating in Sichuan Province, represented by Gengding Pharmacy and Jingyi Hall, is famous for its special processed products such as "Nine-processed Rhei Radix Et Rhizoma (Daihuang)", "Nine-processed Nanxing" and "Prepared Pinelliae Rhizoma (Banxia)", etc. Among which, the more famous product is Linjiang slices (or ripe slices of Aconiti Lateralis Radix Praeparata). The processing method of Linjiang slices is as, wash and clean the drug, mix bile water with clear water, put the monkshood in water, soak for some time, put in a pot, and boil until it is over-heated, after a soak in a moment, take it out and peel, then soak in clean water, then take it out again and cut it into thick slices, then soak again until the color of the surface changed and then steam it in the steaming cage. The firepower needs to be even with no midway turn-off fire. The quality of the slices processed in this way is very good with an oily surface and lustrous. After steaming, the slices should be baked on the roasting mat with medium fire. The products will be ready after drying.

四、京帮的炮制特点

京帮姜制法具有特色，除了姜煮制、姜炒制外，还有姜腌制。姜腌制常用的药材有半夏、天南星和白附子等，通过姜腌制能够较好地降低药材毒性。

盐制法除了盐水炒，还有盐粒炒，即用大青盐粒拌炒药物，适用于质地坚实并入肾经的饮片，如怀牛膝等。

此外，京帮还专门总结了药汁制法的炮制工艺，即以药用液体辅料炮制药物，其中，常用的制辅料包括甘草水煎液、明矾水溶液和黄连水煎液等，通过这些辅料与被炮制药物的有毒成分互相结合，达到降低或消除毒副作用的目的。

京帮在蒸制时多采用铜炖罐，认为这种加热工具传热快并且具有良好的金属稳定性，根据蒸制药物不同，可分为单味药物罐蒸和多味药物罐蒸。北京同仁堂（京帮代表性企业）使用铜炖罐酒蒸制的中药品种包括全鹿丸、参茸卫生丸、乌鸡白凤丸、救苦金丹和安坤赞育丸等，这些成药中的部分药物，强调必须经过酒蒸制方能入药。

京帮中药流派在炮制方法上最具特色的品种包括九转胆星和酒蒸大黄。其中九转胆星制作需 8 年才可完成；酒蒸大黄是将大黄装入铜罐内，倒入定量的绍兴酒蒸制，此法实际为酒炖，与笼屉蒸相比较，炖法可使辅料全部进入药料中，而且气味也不易散失。

Section Four   Processing Technology Characteristics of Jing Society

The methods of processing with ginger in Jing Society are unique, which include not only boiling with ginger, stir-frying with ginger, but also pickling with ginger. The present products processed with ginger pickling are Pinelliae Rhizoma (Banxia), Arisaematis Rhizoma (Tiannanxing), and Typhonii Rhizoma (Baifuzi). Through pickling with ginger, the toxicity of drugs could be reduced better.

Processing drugs with salt is another characteristic method in Jing Society, except stir-frying drugs with saltwater, stir-frying drugs with salt also applied, and the salt is Daqing salt granules, which is suitable for Chinese herbal medicine with solid texture and having the effects on kidney meridian, such as Achyranthis Bidentatae Radix (Huainiuxi).

In addition, in Jing Society, technologies of processing drugs with medicine herbal juice were summarized, that is to use medicine herbal juice to prepare drugs. The commonly used medicine herbal juice includes Glycyrrhizae Radix Et Rhizoma decoction, Alumen solution, and Coptis decoction, etc. The components in medicine herbal juice could combine with the toxic components in drugs to reduce or eliminate the toxic side effects of drugs.

Copper stewing pot is usually used for steaming drugs in processing in Jing Society. It is believed that this heating tool has fast heat transfer and good stability. According to the different natures of drugs, it can be divided into steaming a single drug or several drugs in a pot. The traditional products steamed in copper pots with wine in Tongrentang of Beijing (the representativeness company in Jing Society) include Quanlu pill, Shenrong Weisheng pill, Wuji Baifeng pill, Jiuku Jindan, and Ankun Zanyu pill, etc. Some of these proprietary medicines are emphasized that they must be steamed by wine before they can be used as medicines.

The most distinctive products in Jing Society PCHM include jiuzhuan bile Arisaematis Rhizoma (Tiannanxing) and steamed Rhei Radix Et Rhizoma (Daihuang) with wine. Among them, it takes 8 years to complete the production of jiuzhuan bile Arisaematis Rhizoma (Tiannanxing); the procedure of steaming Rhei Radix Et Rhizoma (Daihuang) with wine is to put Rhei Radix Et Rhizoma into the copper pot, pour quantitative Shaoxing wine and steaming, which is the method of stewing with wine. Comparing to the method of steaming in a cage drawer, steaming in a copper pot can make the drug absorb all the assistant (wine) and avoid the loss of effective components.

五、各流派炮制特点比较

1. 炮制工具的比较

樟帮独特的传统加工炮制工具主要有：铡刀、片刀、刮刀、铁锚、碾槽、冲钵、蟹钳、鹿茸加工壶、压板和硫黄药柜等。尤其是片刀、铡刀面小口薄，轻便锋利，被称为"樟刀"。

建昌帮的切药刀俗称建刀，把长、面大、线直、刃深、吃硬和省力，还可一刀多用，用建刀切制的特色饮片具有斜、薄、大、光的特点，外形精美而实用。由于樟建两帮工具有所不同，古时药学界有"见刀认帮"之说。

建昌帮创制的雷公刨不仅效力高，而且刨的饮片以纵片为多，均匀美观，一直沿用至今。其他的特种工具，如枳壳榨、槟榔榉、香附铲、泽泻笼、茯苓刀、附子筛、麦芽篓、药坛、圆木甑、猪肝色刀石等，各有其用。

京帮在蒸制时多采用铜炖罐，认为这种加热工具传热快且具有良好的金属稳定性，根据蒸制药物不同可分为单味药物罐蒸和多味药物罐蒸。

2. 炮制方法与辅料的比较

樟帮独特的炮制技术闻名遐迩，如特殊发酵工艺炮制的枳壳，皮青、肉厚、色白、香味浓、果囊小、呈凤眼状，质量好且疗效高。在降低饮片毒副作用方面，樟帮也有独特的炮制技艺，如樟帮尿制马钱子（制伏水）、临江片（樟树古称临江，即以姜为辅料，将附子采用特殊蒸制法炮制）等，经炮制后毒性降低的同时提高饮片疗效，以确保高效低毒饮片用于临床。

Section Five   Comparison of Processing Characteristics of Different Schools

1. Comparison of processing tools

The unique traditional processing tools in Zhang Society are as follows: hand hay cutter, blade knife, scraper, iron anchor, mill groove, flushing bowl, crab forceps, deer antler processing pot, pressing board, and sulfur medicine cabinet, etc. Especially the blade knife and hand hay cutter with a small blade, light and sharp, called "zhangdao".

The cutting knife in Jianchang Society is commonly known as "Jiandao", the feature is with a long handle, large, deep, and straight line-like blade, hard and labor-saving. It can also be used as a multi-purpose knife. The characteristic pieces cut by Jiandao are often oblique, thin, large with smooth sections, exquisite and practical appearance. Because of the difference of cutting tools between Zhang Society and Jian Society, there's a saying that "See the knife and you'll know which Society it belongs to".

Leigong planer originated from Jianchang Society is not only effective, and the slices get from Leigong planer are always with lengthwise shape, uniform and beautiful, until now the tool is still used in Jiangchang Society. Other special tools, such as wooden pottery for Aurantii Fructus (Zhike), Iron Betel (Binglang) beech, the Cyperi Rhizoma (Xiangfu) shovel, the Poria (Fuling) knife, screening for Aconiti Lateralis Radix Praeparata (Fuzi), the Hordei Fructus Germinatus (Maiya) basket, the medicine jar for storage, the round wooden steamer for steaming, the auburn color knife stone for sharpening knives, etc., all the tools have their application.

Copper stewing pot is the normally used tool in Jing Society. The tool is considered to have fast heat transfer and good stability. The methods of steaming drugs in copper stewing pot can be divided into steaming a single drug in a pot and steaming several drugs in a pot.

2. Comparisons between processing methods and assistant materials

Zhang Society is famous for its unique processing technology, such as the special fermentation processed Aurantii Fructus (Zhike), which has cyan and thick pericarp, white color, strong fragrance, small fruit sac, and phoenix-eye like shape, with good quality and high curative effect. In the aspect of reducing the side effects of Chinese herbal medicine, there also has unique processing techniques in Zhang Society, such as Strychni Semen (Maqianzi) processed with boy's urine, Linjiang slices (Zhangshu was called Linjiang in ancient times, the method is to use ginger as assistant material, put ginger and Aconiti Lateralis Radix Praeparata-Fuzi together to steam to get prepare aconite), etc. After processing, the toxicity of drugs would be reduced and the curative effect is improved, to ensure the application of high efficiency and low toxicity decoction pieces in the clinic.

樟帮辅料非常讲究，其固体辅料有糙米、蜜麦麸、白矾、豆腐、灶心土、滑石粉、油砂、红糖等。液体辅料有酒、醋、盐水、姜汁、蜜汁、甘草汁、皂角汁、米泔水、米汤、山羊血、猪心血、鳖血、胆汁、羊脂油等。

建昌帮在辅料方面，有选料独特、遵古道地、制备考究、一物多用的特点，其中尤以谷糠作为辅料最具特色，如有谷糠煨、煅制药材，蜜糠炒制多种药材，同时谷糠还用于净选、润制、吸湿、密封养护等，使南糠北麸成为南北药帮炮制流派的一个显著区别。其他辅料，如白矾、朴硝、童便、米泔水、硫黄、砂子等的运用也各有特色。与研究相对较多、较成熟，并已整理出版书籍的樟帮特色炮制技术相比，建昌帮特色的炮制技术，大多是世代口口相传，或老药工根据多年积累的经验，将传统的炮制技艺和炮制理论编成歌诀而代代相传，这对建昌帮炮制技术的传播和推广也起到了一定作用。

川帮炮制技术，具有悠久的传统，以庚鼎药房、精益堂为代表，以九制大黄、九转南星、仙半夏等特色炮制品种闻名。虽然川帮的中药炮制技术具有良好的传统和基础，但由于中医传承的固有规律，一批中药炮制技术也面临着消亡或变异的危险，亟须进一步继承和发扬。

京帮炮制的特点主要体现在炮制方法和辅料特色上。如姜腌制、盐水炒，还有特色的盐粒炒等。京帮善用辅料豆腐，强调用黑豆制作豆腐能更好地降低药物毒性，如以豆腐制附子等。京帮应用米汤的方法独特，专门采用米汤煨制葛根，取其煨制可更好地降低药物燥性。京帮专门总结了药汁制法的炮制工艺，其中常用的药制辅料包括甘草水煎液、明矾水溶液和黄连水煎液等，通过这些辅料与被炮制药物的有毒成分互相结合，达到降低或消除毒副作用的目的。

Zhang Society is very particular about its assistant materials. The solid assistant materials include brown rice, honey wheat bran, alum, tofu, humus flava usta, talcum powder, oil sand, and brown sugar. Liquid assistant materials include wine, vinegar, saltwater, ginger juice, honey juice, Glycyrrhizae Radix Et Rhizoma juice, Gleditsia sinensis juice, water in which rice has been washed, water in which rice has been cooked, goat blood, pig heart blood, turtle blood, bile, mutton oil and so on.

In terms of assistant materials. The characteristics of the processing assistant materials in Jianchang Society include that the selection of assistant materials, the processing methods with assistant materials are unique, authentic, and exquisite, sometimes, the assistant materials are not only used as assistants but can be used in other ways. Among these assistant materials the rice bran is the most special assistant, which is not only used to simmering, calcining and stir-frying drugs, but also can be used for cleaning, lubrication, moisture absorption, sealing and maintenance. "south rice bran north wheat bran" is a significant difference in the processing schools of north and south PCHM gang. Other assistant materials, such as alum, sodium sulfate, boy's urine, water in which rice has been washed, sulfur, sand, etc. also have their characteristics. The study on Zhang Society PCHM is relatively more mature and many research books about Zhang Society PCHM have been published, Compared with Zhang Society PCHM, most of the processing techniques in Jianchang Society are orally transferred or compiled into recipes and passed down from generation to generation. This also has played a certain role in the dissemination and promotion of Jianchang Society PCHM.

The development of Chuan Society PCHM has a long tradition. Chuan Society originated in Sichuan Province, represented by Gengding Pharmacy and Jingyi Hall, is famous for its special processed products such as "Nine-processed Rhei Radix Et Rhizoma (Daihuang)", "Nine-processed Nanxing" and "Prepared Pinelliae Rhizoma Rhizome (Banxia)". The processing technology of traditional Chinese medicine in Chuan Society has a good tradition and foundation. However, due to the inherent law of traditional Chinese medicine inheritance, a batch of traditional PCHM in Chuan Society is also in danger of extinction or variation, which urgently needs further inheritance and development.

The characteristics of processing in Jing Society are mainly in the processing methods and assistant materials, such as pickling with ginger, stir-frying with saltwater, as well as stir-frying with special Daqing salt granules, and so on. Jing Society makes good use of tofu, which is an assistant material in processing. It emphasizes that tofu should come from black beans, which can reduce the toxicity of drugs better, such as processing Aconiti Lateralis Radix Praeparata (Fuzi) with tofu. Water in which rice has been cooked is another special assistant material in Jing Society, which can be used to simmer Pueraria lobate (Gegen) to reduce the dryness of the drug better. In Jing Society, technologies of processing drugs with medicine herbal juice were summed up. The most commonly used medicine herbal juice includes Glycyrrhizae Radix Et Rhizoma decoction, alum solution, and Coptis decoction, etc. The components in medicine herbal juice could combine with the toxic components in drugs to reduce or eliminate the toxic side effects of drugs.

除以上4个全国主流的炮制流派以外，还有山东帮等炮制流派记载，合称十三帮。中药炮制是确保中医药质量的根本保证，有效继承和发扬主流的民间炮制流派技艺，将对我国中医药的发展产生积极影响。

同时，对各炮制流派传统技术特色和优势的传承，将对开展中药炮制技术规范化和产业化研究提供有益启示，为建立稳定可控的技术工艺和饮片质量标准、创新中药炮制技术理念、打造中药饮片产业新前景奠定基础，从而进一步推动我国独有的制药技术传承创新与发展。

In addition to the above four mainstream processing schools in China, there are also other records about the PCHM schools, such as Shandong Society and other Societies, known as Thirteen Societies. PCHM is the fundamental guarantee to ensure the quality of traditional Chinese medicine. Effective inheritance and development of mainstream PCHM techniques will have a positive impact on the development of Chinese medicine.

At the same time, the inheritance of the characteristics and advantages of traditional technology of different processing schools will provide beneficial enlightenment for the research of standardization and industrialization of PCHM, and for the establishment of stable and controllable technological procedure and quality standards of Chinese medicine pieces, the innovation of technological concepts of PCHM, and the creation of new prospects of Chinese medicine pieces industry, which will further to promote the inheritance innovation and development of traditional PCHM.

参考文献：

[1] 郭阿莉.浅谈不同地域中药炮制的特色技术[J].中国民间疗法，2018，26（14）：114-115.

[2] 刘军锋，王红波，张红，等.中药特色炮制技术的帮派特点与发展[J].陕西中医，2019，40（07）：964-967.

[3] 齐玉歌.中药传承任重而道远——中药特色技术传承心得点滴[J].临床医药文献电子杂志，2016，3（47）：9473-9475.

[4] 符颖.不同区域中药炮制特色技术探讨[J].内蒙古中医药，2017，36（20）：82-83.

[5] 龚千锋，易炳学."樟树帮"中药传统炮制特色[N].中国中医药报，2006-09-28（007）.

[6] 周英，李鉴北，欧阳勋志，等.樟树市林下中药经济发展探析[J].江西林业科技，2010（01）：17-19.

[7] 王晓崴，龚千锋.马钱子的炮制沿革、药理作用及安全性的研究进展[J].江西中医药，2013，44（03）：70-72.

[8] 王金权，王娟，樊敏，等.炮制对柴胡质量的影响[J].中医研究，

2011, 24 (05): 43-46.

[9] 张金莲, 谢日健, 刘艳菊, 等. 建昌帮辅料糠的质量标准 [J]. 中国实验方剂学杂志, 2016, 22 (22): 31-33.

[10] 张金莲, 曾昭君, 潘旭兰, 等. 砻糠在建昌帮中药炮制中的应用 [J]. 中草药, 2013, 44 (21): 3092-3094.

[11] 邹红, 童恒力, 孟振豪, 等. 建昌帮特色辅料蜜糠制药的工艺研究 [J]. 时珍国医国药, 2017, 28 (11): 2662-2666.

[12] 孟振豪, 钟凌云. 建昌帮中药炮制概况 [J]. 江西中医药大学学报, 2016, 28 (01): 110-112.

[13] 易炳学, 钟凌云, 龚千锋. 江西建昌帮炙法特色炮制及其现代研究思路 [J]. 时珍国医国药, 2012, 23 (07): 1755-1756.

[14] 曹萍, 梅开丰, 褚小兰, 等. 江西建昌药帮的历史考证 [J]. 江西中医学院学报, 2002 (02): 7-10.

[15] 冯建华，陈秀琼.中药炮制"煨法"考证［J］.时珍国医国药，2004（06）：338-340.

[16] 马艳平.川帮中药特色炮制技术［J］.中医学报，2020，35（08）：1649-1652.

[17] 董震初，徐钰卿，冯祖良.半夏饮片的炮制方法［J］.中药通报，1956（03）：102-104.

[18] 金世元，金艳，李京生锴.金世元谈北京中药用药习惯［J］.首都医药，2011，18（11）：46-47.

[19] 冯守文.京帮炮制拾遗2则［J］.光明中医，2010，25（05）：883-884.

[20] 洪巧瑜，卜训生，李飞，等.以京帮流派中药炮制方法为指导的中药炮制继承教学体系探讨［J］.中国医药导报，2019，16（13）：120-123+131.

第三章　主要常用炮制方法

一、净选加工

净制是中药炮制第一道工序，因为药物在收集过程中会混有沙子，在储存过程中会发生霉变和虫蛀。药物也要选取规定的药用部位，除去非药用部位。

【定义】净选加工是在切制、炮制或调配、制剂前，选取规定的药用部位，除去非药用部位、杂质及霉变品，使其达到药物纯度标准的方法。

【目的】分离药用部位；按照药物大小、粗细进行分档；除去非药用部位；除去杂质。

1. 清除杂质

清除杂质的方法有许多种。每一种除杂方法都可以适用于多种药物，必须根据实际情况灵活选用恰当的方法。根据方法的不同，可分为挑选、筛选、风选和水选等。

（1）挑选：清除混在药物中的杂质及霉变品等，或将药物按大小、粗细等进行分档。将药物放在竹长匾内或摊放在桌上，用手拣去簸不出、筛不下且不能入药的杂质，如核、梗、虫蛀、霉变等部分。

（2）筛选：根据药物和杂质的体积大小不同，选用不规格的筛和罗，以筛去药物中的砂石、杂质，使其达到洁净。筛选的方法使用竹筛、铁丝筛、龟板筛、网筛等。现多用机械操作，主要有震荡式筛药机和小型电动筛药机。后者较适用于有毒、有刺激性及易风化、潮解的药物。

（3）风选：利用药物和杂质的比重不同，借药材起伏的风力，使之与杂质分离的方法。此法主要适用于通过风选可将果柄、花梗、干瘪之物等非药用部位除去的药物。

第二部分 传统炮制

Part II Traditional Processing of Chinese Herbal Medicine

Chapter Three Main Processing Technology

Section One Cleansing

Cleansing is the first process of Chinese medicine processing. The drug may be mixed with sand during the collection process, and mildew and insects will occur during storage. The drug should also be selected from the prescribed medicinal parts and remove non-medicinal parts.

【Definition】Cleansing is a method of selecting a prescribed medicinal part, removing non-medicinal parts, impurities, and mildew products to achieve a drug purity standard before cutting, cannoning or blending, and preparation.

【Purposes】The purposes of cleansing include separating different medicinal parts, classifying drugs according to size and thickness, removing non–medicinal parts and impurities.

1. Removing impurities

There are many ways to remove impurities. As each way applies to different drugs, the proper way should be chosen with flexibility according to the actual situation. These ways include sorting, screening, selection in wind and selection in water, etc.

(1) Sorting: Sorting is to remove impurities and mildewed and rotten materials from the drug, or classify drugs according to size and thickness. Operation methods: Put the raw drugs in a long bamboo plaque or on the table, then pick out the useless impurities that cannot be sifted, such as the nucleus, stems, moth-eaten damages, and mildewed and rotten parts, etc.

(2) Screening: Screening is to sift out sand and impurities by using different sifters according to the shapes and sizes of drugs and impurities. Sand and impurities are sifted out to keep the drugs clean, The screening method uses sifters such as bamboo sifter, iron sifter, tortoise plastron sifter, and net sifter, etc. Nowadays, it is mostly operated by machinery, mainly including oscillating screen medicine machine and small electric screen medicine machine. The latter is more suitable for toxic, irritating, and easily weathered deliquescent drugs.

(3) Selection in wind: Wind selection is a method in which the specific gravity of the drug and the impurities are different, and the wind is undulated by the medicinal material to separate it from the impurities. This method is mainly applicable to drugs that can remove non-medicinal parts such as fruit stalks, peduncles, and dried fruits by air selection.

（4）水选：通过水将药物中附着的泥砂、盐分或不洁之物等杂质选出或漂去的方法。根据药材性质，水选可分为洗净、淘洗和浸漂。

洗净：将药物装在竹筐内，用清水将药材表面的泥土、灰尘、霉斑或其他不洁之物洗去。

淘洗：将药物置于小盛器内，用大量清水荡洗附在药物表面的泥砂或杂质。

浸漂：将药物置于大量清水中浸较长时间，适当翻动，每次换水，至药材毒质、盐分或腥臭异味得以减轻为度。

此外，净制方法还有摘、揉、擦、耷、刷、剪切、挖、剥等。

2. 清除和分离不同药用部位

中药净制是根据原药材情况，结合中医临床用药要求，去根去茎、去枝梗、去皮壳、去毛、去心、去核、去芦、去瓤，去头尾、皮骨、足翅，去残肉，去杂质、霉变品等。

（1）去根去茎：去残根，一般指除去主根、枝根、须根等非药用部位，常用于荆芥、麻黄、黄连等。去残茎，一般指去除非药用部位的残茎，如龙胆草、丹参、续断等。另外，同一类植物根、茎均能入药，但二者作用不同，须分离，分别入药。如麻黄根能止汗，茎能发汗解表，故须分开入药。一般采用剪切、搓揉、风选、挑选等。

（2）去枝梗：指除去某些果实、花、叶类药物的非药用部位，如去除老茎枝、柄蒂，使用量准确。适用于五味子、木兰、栀子等药物。一般采用挑选、切除、摘等方法。

(4) Selection in water: It refers to the method that selecting or removing impurities such as mud, salt, or unclean substances adhering to the drug. According to the nature of the medicinal materials, the water selection can be divided into washing, rinsing, and immersion.

Washing is the way of washing drugs in bamboo baskets, then rinsing away the impurities such as earth, the dust of muddy spots.

Rinsing refers to rinsing drugs in a small container with much water to remove earth and sand or other impurities on the surface of the drug.

Immersing means immersing drugs in the container with much water for a long time, then turning over the drugs properly and changing the water every day to decrease the toxin, salt, and bad odor of the drugs.

There are some other ways of cleansing, such as picking, rubbing, wiping, milling, brushing, cutting with scissors or knife, digging and peeling, etc.

2. Removing and separating different medicinal parts

According to the condition of the original medicinal materials, combined with the requirements of clinical medicine for traditional Chinese medicine, to remove or separate different medicinal parts, such as residual root or stem, bark or testa, hair, the pith of plant, residual parts of the stem, pit, pulp, head, tail, foot and wing, remnant meat, impurities, mold materials, etc.

(1) Removing remnant root or stem: Generally speaking, removing residual root is refer to the removal of non-medicinal parts of herbs, such as taproot, rootlet, fibrous root, etc. It is commonly used in Schizonepetae Herba (Jingjie), Ephedra Herba (Mahuang), Goptidis Rhizoma (Huanglian), etc. Removing residual stem is to remove non–medicinal stems of herbs. It is used in Radix Gentianae (Longdan), Salviae Miltiorrhizae Radix Et Rhizoma (Danshen), Dipsaci Radix (Xuduan), etc.

In addition, If the same type of plant roots and stems can be used as medicine, but the two roles are different, they must be separated and used as medicine. For example, the root and stem of Ephedra Herba (Mahuang) need to be separated because its root has the effect of antiperspirant but its stem has the effect of inducing diaphoresis. Production: remove non–medicinal parts by cutting with scissors, rubbing, selecting in wind or sorting, etc.

(2) Removing stalk: It refers to the removal of non – medicinal parts of fruits, flowers, and leaves to make the dose accurate, such as removing the old stem or the base of the flower or fruit. It is suitable for Schisandrae Chinensis Fructus (Wuweizi), Magnolia liliflora (Mulan), Gardeniae Fructus (Zhizi), etc. Production: remove the non–medicinal parts by selecting, cutting and picking, etc.

（3）去皮壳：药材去皮包括几个方面，有皮类药材去除其栓皮，根及根茎类药材去除其根皮，果实、种子类药材去除其果皮或种皮。去皮壳的目的主要有便于切片，使用量准确，分开药用部位，除去非药用部位等。树皮类药物，如厚朴、黄柏、杜仲可用刀刮去栓皮、苔藓及其他不洁物。有些药物多在产地趁鲜去皮，如知母、桔梗等。果实或种子类药物如草果、砂仁等可砸破皮壳，去壳取仁或可用燀法去皮。

（4）去毛：去毛是去掉药材表面的细绒毛、鳞片及根茎类药材的须根，以防服后刺激咽喉引起咳嗽或其他有害作用，并使药物清洁。某些根茎类药材如骨碎补、香附、知母等表面具毛，须使用砂烫或撞去绒毛的方法去毛。部分叶类药材如枇杷叶、石韦等，须用棕刷刷去绒毛。金樱子果实内部生有淡黄色绒毛，须用工具手工挖尽毛核。其他药物如鹿茸，先用瓷片或玻璃片将其表面绒毛基本刮干净后，再用酒精燃着火将剩余的毛燎焦，注意不能将鹿茸燎焦。

（5）去心："心"指根茎药材的木质部或种子的胚芽。去心包括去根的木质部和枯朽部分、种子的胚等，如地骨皮、五加皮、巴戟天等药材须去心。去心主要有三个目的：第一是去除非药用部位，如巴戟天由于木心所占比重较大且无药效，影响用量的准确性，故要求去除；第二是分离不同的药用部位，如莲子心能清心热、除烦，莲子肉能补脾涩精，故须分别入药；最后是消除药物的副作用，如远志不去心，服之会令人闷。

(3) Removing bark or testa: Removing bark means removing the cork, velamen, fruit peel, or testa of drugs. It is done to facilitate cutting drugs into pieces, making the dose accurate, separating different medicinal parts, and discarding the non-medicinal parts. Cork, moss, and other dirty things can be removed from the bark by scarping barks, such as Magnoliae Officinalis Cortex (Houpo), Phellodendri Chinensis Cortex (Huangbai), and Eucommiae Cortex (Duzhong) with a knife. Barks need to be removed from trees in their habitats when they are still fresh, such as Rhizoma Anemarrhenae (Zhimu) and Radix Platycodi (Jiegeng). Peel or testa need to be removed from some fruit or seed drugs by crushing or scalding, such as Fructus Tsaoko (Caoguo), Fructus Amomi (Sharen).

(4) Removing hair: It means removing fluff, scales on the drug's surface, and fibrous root to avoid irritating throats such as cough or any other side-effects and to make drugs cleaner. coverings need to be cleared from some rhizome drugs by heating with sand or striking, such as Rhizoma Drynariae (Gusuibu), Cyperi Rhizoma (Xiangfu), and Rhizoma Anemarrhenae (Zhimu). Fluff can be removed from some leaf drugs by brushing with coir brush, such as Folium Eriobotryae (Pipaye) and Folium Pyrrosiae (Shiwei). There is flaxen fluff in the inner side of the seeds of Fructus Rosae Laevigatae (Jinyingzi), so hand tools are often used to dig out the fluff and pit. For other drugs, such as Saigae Tataricae Cornu (Lurong), the outside hair needs to be scrapped with ceramic chips or glass sheets. And then burn remnant hair in the fire. Be careful not to burn the drug.

(5) Discarding pith of plant: Pith of plant refers to xylem or embryonic germ of the drugs whose medicinal parts are roots and stems. Discarding pith of plant includes getting rid of the xylem and withered or rotten parts of the stems. For drugs whose medicinal parts are seeds, embryonic germs need to be discarded. The pith of the plant needs to be removed from such drugs as Cortex Lycii (Digupi), Acanthopanax (Wujiapi), and Radix Morindae Officinalis (Bajitian). The purposes of discarding the pith of plant can be summed up into the following three aspects. The first is to remove the non-medicinal parts. Take Radix Morindae Officinalis (Baijitian) as an example, the proportion of xylem is higher and its effect is lower, which may influence the accuracy of the dose in the clinic, so it needs to be discarded. The second is to separate the different medicinal parts. For example, nuts of Semen Nelumbinis (Lianzi) have the effect of clearing heat fire and relieving restlessness, and its pulp can nourish the spleen and astringe sperm, they should be used respectively. The last is to eliminate side-effects, such as Polygalae Radix (Yuanzhi), taking the drugs without discarding the pith of the plant will make patients feel suffocated.

（6）去核：有些果肉类药物，常用果肉而不用核。其中有的核（或种子）属于非药用部位，有些属于药用部位，故须分别用药，如乌梅、山茱萸、山楂、诃子等。去核的目的可按传统的说法总结为的"去核者免滑精"。现代研究认为，去核是因为药物成分含量的差别。到了近代，认为去核的目的是增强药效、保证用药准确以及利于药物有效成分的煎出。去核制作时一般采用风选、筛选、挑选、浸润、切挖等方法。

（7）去芦："芦"指药物的根头、根茎、残茎、残基、叶基等部位。去芦传统的说法是"去芦者免吐"。现代研究未发现人参芦有催吐作用，认为人参没有必要去芦。

（8）去瓤：有些果实类药物，如枳实、枳壳、青皮、木瓜等，须去瓤用于临床。去瓤的目的，传统的说法是"去瓤者免胀"。现代研究认为，去瓤是为了去除非药用部位，以免降低药效，也可以防止药物霉变和虫蛀，又能降低药物的苦酸涩味。

（9）去头尾、皮骨、足翅：部分动物类类药物，为了除去有毒部分或非药用部位，须要去头尾或足翅。如蕲蛇须去头尾，蜈蚣须去头足，斑蝥须去头足翅。去头尾、皮骨，一般采用浸润切除、蒸制剥除等方法。去头足翅，一般采用掰除、挑选等方法。

（10）去残肉：有些动物类药物，如龟甲、鳖甲、动物骨头等，须除去残肉筋膜，以纯净药物。传统的方法一般采用刀刮、挑选、用化学试剂浸漂等。现代可用胰脏净制法和酵母菌净制法。

(6) Removing pit: For some pulp drugs, the pulp instead of the pit is more often used as a medicinal part. Some of these pits (or seeds) are non–medicinal parts, while some are medicinal parts, so different parts should be used respectively. Drugs of this kind include Corni Fructus (Shanzhuyu), Mume Fructus (Wumei), Crataegi Fructus (Shanzha), Chebulae Fructus (Hezi), etc. The purpose of removing the pit is to prevent spermatorrhea in traditional thought. Modern studies believe that it is because the pit has fewer effective components. In modern times, the purpose is thought to improve clinical efficiency, guarantee the accuracy of dispensing drugs and make the effective components easier to be decocted. The methods of selection in wind, screening, sorting, immersing, cutting, and digging are often used in removing the pit.

(7) Removing residual parts of stem: Residual parts of stem refer to the residual parts of the root, rootstalk, stem base, or phytyl group. The purpose is to avoid the side-effect of vomiting in traditional thought. Modern studies have found that there is no vomiting side effect in the residual parts of Panax ginseng (Renshen), so it is unnecessary to discard residual parts of the root of Panax ginseng (Renshen).

(8) Removing pulp: Pulp must be removed from some fruit drugs before they are used in the clinic, such as Fructus Aurantii Immaturus (Zhishi), Fructus Auranti (Zhike), Citri Reticulatae Pericarpium Viride (Qinpi), Fructus Chaenomelis (Mugua). In traditional thought, the purpose of removing pulp is to avoid side–effects of flatulence. Modern studies believe that the purposes of removing pulp are to remove non – medicinal parts so as not to reduce the effect, avoid mildewing and rotting due to insect bites, as well as relieve bitter, sour, and astringent tastes of drugs.

(9) Removing head, tail, skin, bone, foot, and wing: Some animal or insect drugs, to get rid of toxic parts or non – medicinal parts, the head, tail, foot, or wing needs to be removed. For example, head and tail must be removed from Agkistrodon (Qishe); head and feet must be removed from Scolopendra (Wugong); head, feet, and wings must be removed from Mylabris (Banmao). The methods of removing head, tail, skin, and bone include immersing and then cutting, or steaming and then divesting. The method of removing and selecting is generally used.

(10) Removing remnant meat: To purify drugs, remnant meat and fascia must be removed from some animal drugs, such as Carapax et Plastrum Testudinis (Guijia), Carapax Trionycis (Biejia), bones of animals, etc. The traditional methods are to scrape by knife, pick or soak in some chemical reagent. Currently, pancreas enzymolysis and microzyme zymolysis are used to remove the remnant meat efficiently.

二、饮片切制

【饮片的定义】广义而言，凡是直接供中医临床调配处方或中成药生产的所有药物，统称为饮片。狭义而言，饮片是为调配处方而制成的片状药物。

【饮片切制的定义】将净选后的药物软化，切成一定规格的片、丝、块、段等炮制工艺，称为饮片切制。

【目的】便于有效成分的煎出；利于炮制、调配和制剂；便于鉴别和储存。

【分类】切制的方法可分为手切和机器切。

1. 切制前水处理

切制前水处理的目的是使药质地软化，易于切制，同时缓和药性，降低毒性，去除非药用部位，清洁药物。软化药材的原则为"少泡多润，药透水尽"。有些药材在产地趁鲜切制。还有些特殊的软化方法，如黄芩通过蒸制软化，阿胶通过烘烤软化。

（1）常用的水处理方法

淋法：用水淋湿药材，适用于气味芳香和有效成分易随水流失的药材如薄荷、荆芥等。以药材根部软化为度。

淘洗法：淘洗法是用清水洗涤或快速洗涤药物的方法。适用于质地松软、水分易渗入及有效成分易溶于水的药材，如五加皮、甘草、槟榔等，以药物洁净为度。淘洗法还要避免药材"伤水"。现多用洗药机洗涤药材。

泡法：传统的泡法适用于质地坚硬的药材，如木香、乌药等。快速浸泡法适用于质地疏松、柔韧、易潮软的药材，如羌活；含挥发油芳香类药物或含黏液质较多的药物如黄柏等。以完全软化药物为度。操作时，药物要完全浸泡在水中，浸泡的时间尽可能短些，并且视药材质地、水温、季节灵活掌握，药物大小要分档，同时要保留一定的空间。

第二部分　传统炮制

Part II Traditional Processing of Chinese Herbal Medicine

Section Two   Cutting of Prepared Drugs in Pieces

【Definition of decoction pieces】Generally speaking, any drugs used in traditional Chinese medicinal prescription or formulated medicine are called decoction pieces. Narrowly speaking, decoction pieces refer to sliced drugs for Chinese medical prescriptions.

【Definition of cutting of decoction pieces】Cutting of decoction pieces is a kind of processing technology of cutting drugs into specific slices, slivers, chops, sections, etc. after they are cleansed and softened.

【Purposes】The purpose of cutting is to facilitate the decoction of the drugs' effective components, processing, preparation, identification, and storage.

【Classification】The cutting methods can be divided into cutting by hand and cutting by machinery.

1. Processing with water before cutting

The purposes of processing with water before cutting are making drugs soften and easy to cut, moderating drugs' nature and reducing toxicity, cleaning drugs, and discarding non – medicinal parts. The principle of softening drugs is "less soaking, more moistening, penetrating drugs' interior with a proper amount of water". Some drugs should be cut in the habitats when they are fresh. Apart from soaking in water, there are some special methods for softening. For example, Scutellariae Radix (Huangqin) should be softened by steaming; Asini Corii Colla (E'jiao) should be softened by baking.

(1) Common methods of processing with water

Showering: Showering is to shower drugs with water. It is suitable for drugs with fragrant odor and drugs whose effective components are easy to lose with water, such as Menthae Haplocalycis Herba (Bohe), Schizonepetae Herba (Jingjie), etc. The standard is the root becoming soft.

Elutriation (washing): Elutriation is a method of washing or fast lavation with clean water. It is suitable for soft–texture drugs whose effective components are easy to lose with water, such as Cortex Acanthopanics Radicis (Wujiapi), Glycyrrhizae Radix Et Rhizoma (Gancao), Arecae Semen (Binglang), etc. The standard is the cleanness of drugs. Try to avoid using too much water. Currently, drug-washing machines are usually used.

Soaking: Traditional method of soaking is suitable for scleroid drugs, such as Aucklandiae Radix (Muxiang), Radix Linderae (Wuyao), etc. The fast soaking method is suitable for drugs whose texture is loose, soft, and easy to get moist, such as Notopterygii Rhizoma Et Radix (Qianghuo); aromaticity drugs with essential oil and drugs full of phlegmatic temperament such as Angelicae Sinensis Radix (Danggui). The standard is the complete softness of the drug. When processing, immerse the drugs in water thoroughly. Immersing time should be as short as possible, depending on the quality of drugs, temperature of water, and seasons. Classify drugs according to size and remain some room for drug swelling after absorbing water.

漂法：本法适用于有毒性、用盐腌制过的药物及具腥臭异味的药材，如附子、川乌、昆布、紫河车等，以除去其刺激性及咸味、腥臭味为度。

润法：本法适用于质地较坚硬的药材。润的方法有浸润、伏润、露润。浸润适用于质地坚硬的药材，如黄连、木香等；伏润是将水洗的药材在密闭条件下闷润使其软化的方法，适用于质地坚硬的药物，如郁金；露润适用于含糖、脂肪类的药材，如当归、玄参、牛膝等。除此之外，还可采用蒸润、蒸汽喷雾润。

软化有两种改进的方法：真空润药法特点是可以缩短时间，并防止损害药效部位；减压冷浸法可以使水迅速进入药材组织内部，其特点是可提高药材软化的效率。

（2）药材软化程度的检查方法（看水性）

弯曲法：适用于长条状药材，如白芍、山药。

指掐法：适用于团块状药物，如白术、白芷、泽泻等。

穿刺法：适用于粗大块状药物，如大黄。

手捏法：适用于不规则类药材。

剖开法：适合大块规则药材。

2. 切制方法

分为手工切制，机器切制和其他切制。

（1）手工切制：主要有切药刀和片刀。有些特殊的如槟榔可用"蟹爪钳"切，鹿茸可用鹿茸加工壶。

（2）机器切制：主要有剁刀式切药机、旋转式切药机和多功能切药机等。剁刀式切药机主要适用于根、根茎、全草类药材，不适用于颗粒状药材的切制。旋转式切药机一般适用于颗粒类药物和团块类药物，不适合全草类药物。多功能切药机主要适用于块状及根茎、果实类药材，以及多种规格斜形饮片的加工切制。

Rinsing: This method is suitable for toxic drugs, drugs pickled with salt, and drugs with a fishy smell, such as Aconiti Lateralis Radix Praeparata (Fuzi), Aconiti Kusnezoffii Radix (Chuanwu), Laminariae Thallus/Eckloniae Thallus (Kunbu), Placenta hominis (Ziheche), etc. The standard is the disappearance of irritating, salty taste and fishy smell.

Moistening: This method is suitable for hard texture drugs. The methods are immersion, moistening with cover, and moistening without cover. Immersion is suitable for hard texture drugs, such as Goptidis Rhizoma (Huanglian), Aucklandiae Radix (Muxiang), etc. Moistening with cover means covering drugs in a tight container to make them soften. It is also suitable for hard texture drugs, such as Curcumae Radix (Yujin), Chuanxiong Rhizoma (Chuanxiong). Moistening without cover is suitable for drugs with carbohydrate of lipid, such as Angelicae Sinensis Radix (Danggui), Scrophulariae Radix (Xuanshen), Achyranthis Bidentatae Radix (Niuxi), etc. Steaming moistening and steam – spraying moistening can also be used.

There are two ways to improve softening by using a machine. The feature of the vacuum moistening method is to shorten the time and avoid damaging the useful part. Diminution of pressure and cold-soaking method can make water penetrate the interior of the drug quickly and hence improve the efficiency of softening drugs.

(2) Methods of inspecting softening degree

Bending: It is suitable for sliver-type drugs, such as Paeoniae Radix Alba (Baishao) and Dioscoreae Rhizoma (Shanyao).

Pinching with finger: It is suitable for clumping type drugs, such as Atractylodis Macrocephalae Rhizoma (Baizhu), Angelicae Dahuricae Radix (Baizhi), and Alismatis Rhizoma (Zexie).

Puncture: It is suitable for bulky-type drugs, such as Rhei Radix Et Rhizoma (Daihuang).

Pinching with hands: It is suitable for irregular type drugs.

Splitting: It is suitable for large bulk and regular drugs.

2. Cutting methods of prepared drugs in pieces

The methods of cutting include cutting by handwork, machinery, and other methods.

(1) Handwork: It includes Machinery Mince knife and Rotation knife. There are some special tools, such as "clamp cutting" for Arecae Semen (Binglang) nut and processing kettle for Saigae Tataricae Cornu (Lurong).

(2) Machinery: There are Chopping Knife Cutting Machine, Rotary Cutting Machine and Multifunction Cutting Machine and so on. Chopping Knife Cutting Machine is mainly applied to roots, rhizomes, whole plant herbs, not suitable for cutting granular drugs. Rotary Cutting Machine generally applies to the class of grain – like drugs and clump herbs, not suitable for the whole plant drugs. Multifunction Cutting Machine is mainly applied to the roots, bulk herbs and fruits, and a variety of oblique prepared drugs in pieces.

（3）其他切制：镑适用于动物角类切制，如羚羊角等。刨适用于木质或角质坚硬类药材，如檀香、松节等。此外，还有锉、劈、研、磨、打等方法。

3. 饮片干燥

（1）自然干燥

特点：自然干燥的特点是不需特殊设备；适合所有饮片类型；受场地、气候限制；易污染。

分类：阴干适用于芳香类药物，如薄荷，以及具有鲜艳颜色的药物，如红花。晒干适用于黏性大或糖分多的药材，如黄精；粉质类药材，如山药；油质类药材，如当归；部分具有鲜明色泽类药材，如贝母。

（2）人工干燥

特点：人工干燥的特点是干燥快；不受场地、气候限制；清洁卫生；需设备、能源。

设备：包括翻板式干燥机、热风式干燥机、微波干燥技术、太阳能集热干燥技术。

温度：一般药物不超过80℃，含芳香挥发性成分药物一般不超过50℃为宜。

湿度：干燥后的饮片含水量应控制在7%～13%。

注意事项：排出干燥室中的湿气；掌握干燥时间和温度；干燥后冷却；干燥后药材含水量控制在7%～13%。

4. 饮片包装

（1）*饮片包装的作用*：方便饮片的存取、运输、销售；有利于饮片的经营和防止再污染；有利于饮片的美观、清洁、卫生和定期监督检查；有利于促进饮片生产的现代化、标准化；有利于中医饮片临床调配使用；有利于中药饮片的国际贸易。

（2）*饮片包装的方法*：对于贵重、剧毒药材宜用小玻璃瓶、小纸盒分装，并贴上使用说明标签，包装要注重设计和EAN条形码。

(3) Other methods: Pounding is suitable for horny drugs, such as Cornu Saigae Tataricae (Lingyangjiao). Digging is suitable for xylon or horny drugs, such as Lignum Santali Albi (Tanxiang), Lignum Pini Nodi (Songjie), etc. In addition, there are other cutting methods, including rasping, splitting, grinding, striking, etc.

3. Dryness of prepared drugs in pieces

(1) Air drying

Features: Special equipment is not needed for air drying. And it is suitable for all types of prepared drugs in pieces, but limited by the place and climate, and easy to be contaminated.

Classification: Drying in shade is suitable for drugs containing fragrant components, such as Menthae Haplocalycis Herba (Bohe) and drugs with beautiful color. Flos Carthami (Honghua) is an example. Drying in the sunshine is suitable for viscidity drugs containing saccharic, such as Rhizoma Polygonati (Huangjing); powdery drugs, such as Dioscoreae Rhizoma (Shanyao); oiliness drugs, such as Angelicae Sinensis Radix (Danggui); color and luster drugs, such as Bulbus Fritillaria (Beimu).

(2) Artificial drying

Features: The features of artificial drying are quick-drying; not limited by place and climate; neat and clean; in need of equipment and energy.

Equipment: They are mainly the inverted plate drying machine, hot air dryer, microwave drying technology, and solar collector drying technology.

Temperature: The temperature for normal drugs should be less than 80 ℃, while for drugs containing fragrant components, the temperature should be less than 50 ℃.

Moisture content: The moisture content of the prepared drug in pieces after drying should be between 7% and 13%.

Notices: The notices include removing dampness in the drying room before drying, controlling the time and temperature of drying, cooling the drugs after drying, and making sure the moisture content after drying is between 7% and 13%.

4. Packing of prepared drugs in pieces

(1) Functions: It can facilitate storage, transportation, and selling. It helps to improve the drugs' sales and avoid drugs being contaminated again. It makes prepared drugs in pieces beautiful, clean and hygienic, and easy for regular supervision and inspection. It promotes modernization and standardization of the production of decoction pieces. It is beneficial for clinical prescriptions. It facilitates international trade of prepared drugs in pieces of TCM.

(2) Notices of packing: Precious and toxic drugs are better stored in small glass bottles and paper boxes with instruction labels. Pay attention to decoration and EAN code of packing.

5. 饮片类型

（1）饮片类型及规格

极薄片：厚度为 0.5mm，如羚羊角。

薄片：厚度为 1～2mm，如白芍。

厚片：厚度为 2～4mm，如茯苓。

斜片：厚度为 2～4mm，瓜子片（如桂枝），马蹄片（如大黄），柳叶片（如甘草）。

直片：厚度为 2～4mm，如何首乌。

丝：细丝 2～3mm，如黄柏；粗丝 5～10mm，如厚朴。

段：长为 10～15mm，如薄荷。

块：8～12mm³，如阿胶。

（2）**切制方法**：分为横切、顺切、斜切。

（3）切制原则

按药效部位：根、根茎类药材宜切片；角类宜切制极薄片、粉。

按质地和形状：质地致密、结实者宜切薄片，质地松泡、粉性大者宜切厚片，形体大、组织致密宜切直片，长条形宜切斜片。

6. 不良因素对饮片质量的影响

（1）**败片**：在中药饮片切制过程中所有不符合切制规格、片形标准的饮片，都称为败片。主要包括连刀片、掉边与炸心片、皱纹片等。

连刀片：是饮片之间相牵连、未完全切断的现象。系药物软化时，外部含水量过多，或刀具不锋利所致。

掉边与炸心片：是药材切断后，饮片内外相脱离或药材破碎的现象。系药材软化时内外软硬度不同所致。

皱纹片：是饮片切面粗糙，具鱼鳞样斑痕的现象。系药材软化时水性不及，或刀具不锋利所致。

（2）**翘片**：饮片边缘卷曲而不平整。系药材软化时，内部含水分过多所致。

（3）**变色与走味**：指饮片干燥后失去原药材的色泽或失去原有的气味。系药材软化时浸泡时间太长，或干燥地方选用不当所致。

5. Types

(1) Types and sizes

Extremely thin slice: 0.5mm, such as Saigae Tataricae Cornu (Lingyangjiao)

Thin slice: 1~2mm, such as Paeoniae Radix Alba (Baishao).

Thick slice: 2~4mm, such as Poria (Fuling).

Oblique slice: 2~4mm, such as Cinnamomi Ramulus (Guizhi), Rhei Radix Et Rhizoma (Daihuang), Glycyrrhizae Radix Et Rhizoma (Gancao).

Straight slice: 2~4mm, such as Polygoni Multiflori Radix (Heshouwu).

Sliver thin sliver: 2~3mm, such as Phellodendri Chinensis Cortex (Huangbai) wide sliver 5~10mm, such as Magnoliae Officinalis Cortex (Houpo).

Section: 10~15mm, such as Menthae Haplocalycis Herba (Bohe).

Chop: 8~12mm^3, such as Asini Corii Colla (E'jiao).

(2) Cutting ways: The main ways of cutting include vertical cutting, cross-section cutting, and titled cutting.

(3) Principle

According to their different medicinal parts: root and rhizome drugs should be cut into slices; and horny drugs should be cut into extremely thin slices or powder.

According to their different texture and shape: hard pykno – texture drugs should be cut into thin slices, while drugs of rarefaction and brittleness should be cut into thick slices; large and pykno – texture drugs should be cut into straight slices, while sliver drugs can be cut into oblique slices.

6. Adverse influences on the quality of prepared drugs in pieces

(1) Failed Pieces: Failed pieces refer to all the pieces that don't meet the specification standards of cutting, including unbroken pieces, fringe or center fallen pieces, wrinkle pieces, etc.

Unbroken pieces: They refer to unbroken pieces between adjacent intersections. It is due to too much water in the drugs when they are being softened or dull cutting knife.

Fringe or centre fallen pieces: They refer to the center part and fringe of pieces separated or broken. It is due to different hardness between different parts of the drugs after they are being softened.

Wrinkle pieces: They refer to rough sections with fish scales – like phenomenon. It is due to inadequate water when the drugs are being softened or dull cutting knife.

(2) Curling pieces: The cut pieces are curling and uneven showing on the surface of prepared drugs in pieces. It is due to too much water inside the drugs when they are being softened.

(3) Allochromasia and palling: It refers to the loss of luster and smell of the original drugs after they are dried. It is due to the too long time of soaking or improper storing place for drying.

（4）走油：是药材或饮片表面有油分或黏液质渗出的现象。系药材软化时吸水量太过或环境温度过高所致。

（5）发霉：在适宜的温度和湿度条件下，因为霉菌的繁殖生长，在饮片及其炮制品表面布满菌丝的现象。

7. 其他加工

（1）研磨：适用于矿物类药，如自然铜；贝壳类药，如穿山甲；果实或种子类药，如栀子；小型块茎，如贝母。目的是利于有效成分的煎出，便于调配处方。

（2）制绒：麻黄可通过制成麻黄绒来减缓其作用。

（3）拌衣：青黛和朱砂可作拌衣常用辅料，如青黛拌灯心草、朱砂拌茯苓等，可增强药效。

（4）揉搓：竹茹和谷精草可用制绒法进行炮制，便于调剂、制剂。

三、炒法

【定义】将净制或切制过的药物置炒制容器内不断翻动或转动，或先将辅料加热，然后加入药物进行加工炮制的方法。

【分类】可分为清炒法和加辅料炒法。清炒法可分为炒黄、炒焦、炒炭法；加辅料炒法可分为麦麸炒、米炒、土炒、砂炒、蛤粉炒和滑石粉炒等。

【工艺】将净制或切制过的药物，筛去灰屑，大小分档，置于预热过的炒制容器内，加辅料或不加辅料，用不同火力加热，并不断翻动或转动使之达到一定程度，主要操作方法有手工炒和机器炒。手工炒制的优点是所需仪器简单，适合于小规模生产，而机器炒制则更适用于大规模生产。其操作要点如下：最好使用斜锅，利于搅拌和翻动；适合于加工炮制少量多种类的药物。

(4) Extensive diffusion of Oil: It refers to the greasy surface or exuding mucus. It is due to too much water absorbed when the drugs are the softened or too high temperature of the environment.

(5) Mildewing: It refers to tiny fungus forming mycelium coating on the prepared drugs in pieces at the appropriate temperature and in damp conditions.

7. Other processing methods

(1) Grinding: Grinding is suitable for minerals, such as Pyritum (Zirantong) and shell drugs like Squama Manis (Chuanshanjia), fruits, and seeds, such as Gardeniae Fructus (Zhizi), small shape tuber, such as Bulbus Fritillaria (Beimu). The purposes of grinding are to facilitate the dissolution of effective components and make prescription and preparation easy.

(2) Fine hair making: Ephedrae Herba (Mahuang) could be made into ephedrae fine hair to moderate its effects.

(3) Mix with adjuvant materials: Indigo Naturalis (Qingdai) and Cinnabaris (Zhusha) can be often used as adjuvant materials, such as Indigo Naturalis (Qingdai) mixed with Junci Medulla (Dengxincao) and Cinnabaris (Zhusha) mixed with Poria (Fuling), to improve the efficacy of drugs.

(4) Malaxation: This method can be used to process Bambusae Caulis in Taeniam (Zhuru) and Eriocauli Flos (Gujingcao) to facilitate prescription and preparation.

Section Three Stir-frying

【Definition】Stir–frying refers to the processing method that stirs and rotates the cleansed or drugs in pieces in a frying container constantly if stir-frying with adjuvant materials, preheating the adjuvant materials before processing with the drugs.

【Classification】The method of stir–frying can be divided into stir–frying with adjuvant materials and stir–frying without adjuvant materials. ① Stir–frying without Adjuvant MaterialsStir–bake to yellow is a processing method of heating the drugs with slow or medium fire until they turn yellow or deeper in color outside, or the drugs swell or explode to release the intrinsic odor. Stir–bake to brown is a processing method of stir-frying the drugs with medium or strong fire until the surface of the drugs appears light brown or coke brown. Stir–bake to charcoal is a processing method of stir-frying the drugs with strong or medium fire until the surface of the drugs appears to coke brown or black. ② Stir – Frying with Adjuvant Materials: It can be divided into wheat bran stir-frying, rice stir-frying, earth stir-frying, sand stir-frying, clam meal stir-frying, and talcum powder stir-frying.

【Technics】The cleansed or cut drugs are first screened to remove ashes and separated by size. Then they are put into a preheated container. Adding adjuvant materials or not, the drugs are stirred or rotated constantly with different fire levels until they reach the desired degree. This processing can be achieved by handwork or machine. The advantage of stir-frying by handwork is the simple equipment which is suitable for small-scale production. For mass processing, stir-frying by machine would be the better choice. The main points of operation are as follows: It is best to use a slanting pot to facilitate agitation and flipping; it is suitable for processing a small variety of drugs.

1. 清炒法

（1）炒黄法

定义：将净制或切制过的药物，置于炒制容器内，用文火或中火加热，并不断翻动或转动，使药物表面呈黄色或颜色加深，或发泡鼓起，或爆裂，并逸出固有气味的方法。

目的：增强疗效；降低毒性或副作用。

工艺：将净制或切制过的药物，筛去灰屑，大小分档，置于预热过的炒制容器内，不加辅料，用不同火力加热，并不断翻动或转动使之达到一定程度。

判断标准：断面呈淡黄色；颜色加深；有爆鸣声；外观形态改变（发泡鼓起）；爆裂；逸出固有气味。

注意事项：当药物炒至淡黄色时，注意避免炒焦。通常使用文火加热，而对一些特殊药材可使用中火进行加热，如苍耳子、王不留行、牛蒡子、薏苡仁等。

适用药物：果实类与种子类药材适用炒黄法进行炮制，某些根茎类或者是动物药也使用此法进行炮制，如赤芍、槐花、九香虫和海螵蛸。

（2）炒焦法

定义：将净选或切制后的药物，置于炒制容器内，用中火或武火加热，炒至药物表面呈焦黄或焦褐色。

目的：增强药物消食健脾的功效，如麦芽、谷芽和神曲；减少药物的刺激性，如槟榔、栀子和川楝子。

工艺：将净制或切制过的药物，筛去灰屑，大小分档，置于预热过的炒制容器内，不加辅料，用不同火力加热，并不断翻动或转动使之达到一定程度。

判断标准：药物表面呈焦黄或焦褐色，内部焦黄，如山楂和神曲；药物表面呈焦黄色，内部颜色加深，如谷芽。

1. Stir-frying without adjuvant materials

(1) Stir–bake to yellow

Definition: Stir-bake to yellow is a processing method that stirs and rotates the cleansed or cut drugs with slow or medium fire in a frying container constantly until the surface of the drugs appears yellow or deeper in color.

Purposes: Improve the drugs' efficacy. Reduce the drugs' toxicity or side effects.

Technics: Screened out ashes and separated by size, the cleansed or cut drugs are put into a preheated container. Without adding any adjuvant materials, the drugs are heated with different fire levels and stirred or rotated constantly until they reach the desired degree.

Standards: The cutting surface turns yellowish. Color is deepened. The sound of crack could be heard. The shapes of drugs are changed or swelled. Exploding. The intrinsic odor is released.

Notices: When the color of the drugs turns yellowish, over-frying should be avoided. It is usually heated with slow fire while the medium fire also can be used for some special drugs. Such as Xanthii Fructus (Cang'erzi), Vaccariae Semen (Wangbuliuxing), Arctii Fructus (Niubangzi), and Coicis Semen (yiyiren).

Suitable drugs for application: Drugs made from fruits and seeds are usually processed with this method. But some drugs made from rhizomes or even animals could also be processed with this method, such as Paeoniae Radix Rubra (Chishao), Sophorae Flos (Huaihua), Aspongopus (Jiuxiangchong), and Sepiae Endoconcha (Haipiaoxiao).

(2) Parching

Definition: It is a processing method of stir-frying the cleansed or cut drugs with medium or strong fire until they are parched.

Purposes: Strengthen the drugs' effects of fortifying the spleen and promoting digestion. Hordei Fructus Germinatus (Maiya), Setariae Frucuts Germinatus (Guya), and Massa Medicata Fermanetata (Shenqu) are good examples. Moderate the nature of drugs and reduce the irritating nature of drugs. Such as Arecae Semen (Binglang), Gardeniae Fructus (Zhizi) and Toosendan Fructus (Chuanlianzi).

Technics: Screened out ashes and separated by size, the cleansed or cut drugs are put into a preheated container. Without adding any adjuvant materials, the drugs are heated with different fire levels and stirred or rotated constantly until they reach the desired degree.

Standards: For the drugs such as Crataegi Fructus (Shanzha) and Massa Medicata Fermentata (Shenqu), the color turns coke brown outside and coke yellow inside. For the drugs such as Crataegi Fructus (Shanzha) and Setariae Frucuts Germinatus (Guya), the color turns coke yellow outside and a deeper color inside.

注意事项：当炒焦药物时，注意避免炭化。

适用药物：适用炒焦法进行炮制的药物多具健脾养胃之功效，对肠胃造成刺激的药物也可用此法进行炮制。

（3）炒炭法

定义：用武火或中火加热药物，炒至其炭化，表面焦黑色或焦褐色。

目的：增强或产生止血作用，如地榆和蒲黄；增强药物的止泻作用，如乌梅炭和石榴皮炭。

工艺：将净制或切制过的药物，筛去灰屑，大小分档，置预热过的炒制容器内，不加辅料，用不同火力加热，并不断翻动或转动使之达到一定程度，并喷淋少许清水灭尽火星。

判断标准：炒至药物表面焦黑色或焦褐色，如根与块茎类药物；达到"炒炭存性"的要求，如花、叶和全草类药物；药物表面呈黑色且具有光泽，如茜草等。

注意事项：操作时要掌握好火力，质地坚实的药物宜用武火，质地疏松的花、花粉、叶、全草类药物可用中火，视具体药物灵活掌握；须喷淋适量清水灭尽火星，以免引起燃烧；炒炭要求存性；药物必须在晾凉之后贮藏，避免复燃。

适用药物：此法适用于具有止血、止泻作用的药物。

2. 加固体辅料炒法

（1）麸炒法

定义：将净制或切制后的药物用麦麸熏炒至一定程度的方法，通常使用中火炒制。

目的：降低挥发油的含量；加热药物；使炮制过程有充足的时间或热量；矫臭矫味；增强药物补气和中、涩肠止泻之功效。

工艺：先用中火或武火将锅烧热，再将麦麸均匀撒入热锅中，至起烟时投入药物，快速均匀翻动，炒至药物表面呈黄色，麦麸变黑时取出。

辅料用量：每100kg药物，用麦麸10～15kg。

Notices: When stir-frying the drugs to be parched, avoid being charred.

Suitable drugs for application: Drugs that have the functions of fortifying the spleen to promote digestion can be processed with this method. And drugs that irritate intestines and stomach also can be stir-fried to be parched.

(3) Carbonizing by stir-frying

Definition: It is a method of stir-frying the drugs to a carbonized state with strong or medium fire.

Purposes: Strengthen or bring the drugs' effect of hemostasis. Sanuisorbae Radix (Diyu) and Typhae Pollen (Puhuang) are good examples. Strengthen the drugs' effect of arresting diarrhea. Mume Fructus (Wumei) and Granati Pericarpium (Shiliupi) are good examples.

Technics: Screened out ashes and separated by size, the cleansed or cut drugs are put into a preheated container. Not adding any adjuvant materials, the drugs are heated with different fire levels and stirred or rotated constantly until they reach the desired degree. Then spray some water to extinguish sparkles.

Standards: For the drugs made from roots and tubers, stir–fry them until the drugs turn coke black or coke brown outside. For the drugs made from flowers or leaves and herbs, stir–fry them until "burned as charcoal while function preserved". For the drugs such as Indian Rubiae Radix Et Rhizoma (Qiancao), stir–fry them until the drugs turn black and burnished.

Notices: Different fire levels should be applied according to different drugs. For example, a strong fire should be used to heat drugs with hard texture, while a medium fire can be applied to heat drugs with soft texture such as drugs made from flower, pollen, leaf, or grass. Spray water to extinguish sparkles to avoid the drugs being burnt thoroughly. The functions of drugs should be preserved when they are carbonized by stir-frying. Store after being cooled to avoid recrudescence.

Suitable drugs for application: The method can be used to process drugs with effects of hemostasis and arresting diarrhea.

2. Stir-frying with adjuvant materials

(1) Stir-frying with wheat bran

Definition: It is a method of stir-frying the cleansed or cut drugs with wheat bran, usually with medium fire.

Purposes: Reduce the content of volatile oil. Heat the drugs. Provide sufficient time or heat in processing. Remove the bad odor and modify the drugs' taste. Strengthen the drug's effects of tonifying qi and harmonizing the center, astringing the intestines, and checking diarrhea.

Technics: Preheat a pan with medium or strong fire and sprinkle the bran into it evenly. Add the drugs in when the bran smokes and stir – fry them together quickly until the drugs become yellow and the bran turns black.

Amount of Adjuvant Material: Use 10~15kg wheat bran per 100kg drugs.

注意事项：使用中火对锅进行预热；麦麸要均匀撒布热锅中；麸炒药物要求干燥；麸炒药物达到标准时要求迅速出锅。

适用药物：常用麦麸炒制能补脾胃或作用强烈、有腥味的药物。

（2）米炒法

定义：将净制或切制后的药物与米同炒至一定程度的方法，一般使用中火加热。

目的：吸附药物的毒性成分；增强药物的健脾止泻作用。

工艺：先将锅烧热，加入定量的米，用中火炒至冒烟时，投入药物，快速拌炒至药物表面颜色加深，米呈焦黄或焦褐色，取出。

辅料用量：每100kg药物，用米20kg。

注意事项：炮制昆虫类药物时，一般以米的色泽观察火候；炮制植物类药物时，观察药物色泽变化。

适用药物：毒性药物，如斑蝥；具有补脾益气作用的药物，如党参。

（3）土炒法

定义：将净制或切制后的药物与灶心土同炒至一定程度的方法，一般使用中火加热。

目的：能增强补脾止泻的功能。

工艺：将灶心土研成细粉，置于锅内，用中火加热，炒至土呈灵活状态时投入净药物，翻炒至药物表面均匀挂上一层土粉，并透出香气时，取出。

辅料用量：每100kg药物，用土粉25～30kg。

适用药物：具有补脾止泻功能的药物。

（4）砂炒法

定义：将净制或切制后的药物与热砂用武火加热，同炒至一定程度的方法。

目的：便于调剂和制剂；便于去毛；降低毒性；矫臭矫味。

Notices: Preheat the pan with medium fire. Sprinkle the bran evenly. Dry the drugs before processing. Take the drugs out quickly when they are stir-fried to the desired degree.

Suitable drugs for application: This method can be used to process drugs with the effect of tonifying the spleen and stomach, or drugs with strong effects and fishy odor.

(2) Stir-frying with rice

Definition: It is a method of stir-frying the cleaned and cut drugs with rice to a certain degree, usually with medium fire.

Purposes: Absorb the toxic components. Strengthen the effect of fortifying the spleen and arresting diarrhea.

Technics: Put the rice into a preheated pan first and heat with medium fire until the rice smokes. Then add drugs into the pan and stir quickly until the drugs' color turns deeper or the rice's color becomes coke yellow or coke brown.

Amount of Adjuvant Material: Use 20kg rice for 100kg drugs.

Notices: When processing insect drugs, pay attention to the color change of the rice. When processing plant drugs, pay attention to the color change of the drug.

Suitable drugs for application: This method can be used to process toxic drugs (Mylabris-Banmao) and drugs with the effect of tonifying the spleen and boosting qi (Codonopsis Radix-Dangshen).

(3) Stir-frying with soil

Definition: It is a method of stir-frying the cleaned or cut drugs with soil to a certain degree, normally with medium fire.

Purposes: Processing with soil can strengthen the effects of tonifying the spleen and arresting diarrhea.

Technics: Grind the soil and put it into a pan, heating with medium fire. Stir – fry the soil to be loose and smooth. Add the drugs in and stir – fry them together until the drugs' surface is evenly covered with soil. When there is an aroma, take them out and screen out the soil.

Amount of adjuvant material: 25~30kg soil for 100kg drugs.

Suitable drugs for application: This method can be used to process drugs with the effects of tonifying the spleen and arresting diarrhea.

(4) Stir-frying with sand

Definition: It is a method of stir-frying the cleaned or cut drugs with hot sand to a certain degree, usually heating with strong fire.

Purposes: Help compounding and preparing. Facilitate removing the hair of the drug. Reduce toxicity. Modify the bad taste and odor.

工艺：取制过的砂置于锅内，用武火加热至灵活状态、容易翻动时，投入药物，不断用砂掩埋、翻动，至质地酥脆或鼓起，外表呈黄色或较原色加深时取出，趁热投入醋中略浸，取出，干燥即得。

辅料用量：以能掩盖所加药物为度。

注意事项：药物在炮制之前须经干燥处理；砂炒温度要适中；翻动要勤，成品出锅要快，出锅后尽快除去砂；有时可在砂中加入植物油使其更加灵活，油砂可反复使用。

适用药物：适用于质地坚硬或具有毒性的药物。

（5）蛤粉炒法

定义：将净制或切制后的药物与蛤粉用中火加热，同炒至一定程度的方法。

辅料用量：每100kg药物，用蛤粉30～50kg。

注意事项：药物须大小分档，分别炒制；炒制时火力不宜过大；胶丁下锅翻炒要速度快而均匀；辅料须经常更换；贵重、细料药物在大批炒制前采取试投的方法，以便掌握火力，保证炒制品质量。

适用药物：胶类药物。

（6）滑石粉炒法

定义：将净制或切制后的药物与滑石粉用中火加热，同炒至一定程度的方法。

辅料用量：每100kg药物，用蛤粉40～50kg。

适用药物：韧性较大的动物类药物。

四、炙法

【定义】将净选或切制后的药物，加入一定量的液体辅料拌炒，使辅料逐渐渗入药物组织内部的炮制方法。

Technics: Put the processed sand into a pan and heat it with strong fire until the sand becomes smooth and easy to be rotated. Add drugs in and stir – fry them together constantly to let the drugs be covered by the sand. Take the drugs out when they swell, turn crisp in texture and yellow or deeper in color outside. Or put the drugs into vinegar for a short while when they are still hot, then take them out for drying.

Amount of adjuvant material: The adjuvant material should cover the drug.

Notices: Drugs should be dried before processing. The temperature should be controlled. The drugs should be stir-fried frequently. Take the drugs out and screen out the sand immediately when they are ready. Sometimes plant oil can be added to sand to make it smooth enough. The sand with oil can be used repeatedly.

Suitable drugs for application: Suitable drugs for this method are drugs with hardy texture or toxicity.

(5) Stir-frying with clam powder

Definition: It is a method of stir-frying the cleaned or cut drugs with clam powder to a certain degree, normally with medium fire.

Amount of adjuvant material: Use 30~35kg clam powder for 100kg drugs.

Notices: Stir – fry the drugs separately according to their size. Do not use too strong fire while processing. Stir – fry drugs quickly and evenly in the pan. Change the adjuvant materials frequently. Use a few drugs to test the temperature before a great amount of valuable and slight drugs are being processed.

Suitable drugs for application: Suitable drugs are mastic drugs.

(6) Stir-frying with talcum powder

Definition: It is a method of stir-frying the cleaned or cut drugs with Talcum powder to a certain degree, normally with medium fire.

Amount of adjuvant material: Use 40~50kg Talcum powder for 100kg drugs.

Suitable drugs for application: Suitable drugs are animal drugs with strong tenacity.

Section Four   Stir-frying with Liquid Adjuvant Material

【Definition】Stir – frying with liquid adjuvant materials refers to the processing method that stir-fries purified or cut drugs with some liquid adjuvant materials so that the auxiliary material gradually infiltrates into the inside of the drug tissue.

【分类】炙法根据所用辅料不同,可分为酒炙(大黄)、醋炙(甘遂)、盐炙(黄柏)、姜炙(厚朴)、蜜炙(麻黄)、油炙(三七)等法。

【炙法与加固体辅料炒法的区别】加固体辅料炒法与加液体辅料炒法在一些方面有所区别,如下表:

	液体辅料	固体辅料
温度	文火	中火或武火
时间	长	短
过程	渗透入药物	不渗透入药物
性质	大多数药物的理化性质发生改变	热传导,增强药效,使药物表面颜色加深
操作方法	先对药物进行炒制,然后加入辅料;或者先将药物与辅料拌匀,然后进行炒制	先对辅料进行加热,然后加入药物

【Classification】According to different adjuvant materials, stir-frying could be classified into the following concrete methods, i.e.:

stir-frying with wine, such asRhei Radix Et Rhizoma (Daihuang).

stir-frying with vinegar, such as Kansui Radix (Gansui).

stir-frying with saltwater, such as Phellodendri Chinensis Cortex (Huangbai).

stir-frying with ginger juice, such as Magnoliae Officinalis Cortex (Houpo).

stir-frying with refined honey, such as Ephedrae Herba (Mahuang).

and stir-frying with oil, such as Notoginseng Radix Et Rhizoma (Sanqi).

【Differences between stir-frying with liquid and solid adjuvant materials】In some aspects, there are differences between stir-frying with solid dajuvant materials and liquid adjuvant materials. The differences are as follows:

	Liquid Adjuvant Materials	**Solid Adjuvant Materials**
Temperature	Low	Medium or high
Time	Long	Short
Process	Adjuvant materials penetrating drugs	Adjuvant materials not penetrating drugs
Nature	Adjuvant materials make most drugs' physico–chemical properties change	As heat transfer, adjuvant materials strengthen effects and deepen the superficial color of drugs
Operation	Fry drugs first, then add adjuvant materials or evenly mix adjuvant materials with drugs first, then fry	Heat the adjuvant materials first, then add drugs

1. 酒炙法

定义：将净选或切制后的药物，加入一定量的酒，用文火拌炒至一定程度的方法。

目的：①改变药性。例如，龙胆主要功效为清热泻火燥湿，但是经过酒炙之后，则用于肝胆实火所致的头胀、头痛及目赤肿痛。②协同作用。经过炮制之后，药物活血通络的作用得到增强，如当归。③改变药性。经过炮制之后，药物的寒凉之性能得以缓和，如黄连。④提高药物有效成分的溶出率。药物经过炮制，其有效成分溶出率增大，增强了疗效，如黄芩。⑤矫臭去腥。一些具有腥气的动物类药物，经过炮制后可除去或减弱腥臭气，如乌梢蛇。⑥降低药物的毒副作用，并使其质地坚硬易于粉碎，如蟾酥。

工艺：①先拌酒后炒药。适用于大多数药物，特别使用于质地较坚实的根茎类药物。将净制或切制后的药物与一定量的酒拌匀，稍闷润，待酒被吸尽后，置于炒制容器内，用文火炒干。②先炒药后加酒。适用于质地疏松的药物，如五灵脂。先将净制或切制后的药物，置于炒制容器内，加热至一定程度，再喷洒一定量的酒炒干。

辅料用量：一般每 100kg 药物，用黄酒 10～20kg。

适用药物：性质苦寒的药物，如大黄；活血祛瘀的药物，如当归；祛风通络的药物，如威灵仙。

1. Stir-frying with wine

Definition: Stir-frying with wine refers to the processing method that stir-fries purified or cut drugs with a certain amount of wine, and stir-fries them with mild fire to a certain degree.

Purposes: ① Change drugs' properties. For example, the main effects of Gentianae Radix Et Rhizoma (Longdan) are to clear heat, purge fire, and dry dampness. But after being stir-fried with wine, the main effects are changed to treat headache, swelling, and pain of the eye due to the pathogenic fire of the liver and gallbladder. ② Synergistic effect. After being processed, the drugs' effect of promoting blood flow to unblock collateral will be strengthened, such as Angelicae Sinensis Radix (Danggui). ③ Moderate drugs' properties. After being processed, the cold property of some drugs will be moderated, such as Goptidis Rhizoma (Huanglian). ④ Increase the dissolution rate of the effective components of drugs. After being processed, the dissolution rate of the effective components would be increased, the effect will be improved, such as Scutellariae Radix (Huangqin). ⑤ Modify the smell and stink of some drugs. After being processed, the bad smell and stink of some animal drugs will be removed or reduced, such as Zaocys (Wushaoshe). ⑥ Reduce drugs' toxicity or side – effects, and make their texture crisp and easy to be crushed, such as Bufonis Venenum (Chansu).

Technics: There are two kinds of processing technologies. ① Mix wine with drugs firstly and then fry. The way is suitable for most drugs, especially for drugs with hard texture tuber. Mix the cleaned or cut drugs with wine evenly until they are slightly moistened, put the drugs into a frying container after the wine is absorbed thoroughly, then fry with a mild fire until the drugs become dry. ② Fry drugs firstly and then sprinkle wine on the drugs' surface. The way is suitable for those drugs with a crisp texture, such as Faeces Togopteri (Wulingzhi). Put the cleaned or cut drugs into a frying container, and heat it to some degree, then spray some wine evenly on the drugs' surface and fry them to make them dry.

Amount of adjuvant material: The amount of the liquid adjuvant materials needed in the procedures of stir-frying with wine is 10~10kg yellow wine per 100kg drugs.

Suitable drugs for application: Suitable for drugs with bitter and cold nature, such as Angelicae Sinensis Radix (Daihuang). Suitable for drugs with the effect of promoting blood flow to eliminate blood stasis, such as Angelicae Sinensis Radix (Danggui). Suitable for drugs with the effect of expelling wind and removing collaterals, such as Clematidis Radix Et Rhizoma (Weilingxian).

2. 醋炙法

定义：将净选或切制后的药物，加入定量米醋低温拌炒至规定程度的方法。

目的：①引药入肝，增强活血理气止痛作用。如柴胡醋炙后能增强疏肝止痛的作用；延胡索醋炙后能增强活血散瘀的作用。②降低毒性，缓和药性。如芫花经醋炙之后，可消减毒性，缓和峻下作用。③矫臭矫味。如乳香经醋炙后可减少其不良气味。④使药物易于粉碎和有效成分的溶出。如矿物药（自然铜）和贝类（龟甲）经过炮制之后，其质地由坚硬变为酥脆。

工艺：①先拌醋后炒药。将净制或切制后的药物，加入定量米醋拌匀，闷润，待醋被吸尽后，置于炒制容器内，用文火炒至一定程度，取出晾凉即得。此法适用于大多数药物。②先炒药后喷醋。将净选后的药物，置于炒制容器内，文火炒至规定程度，喷洒定量米醋，炒至微干，取出后继续翻动，摊开晾凉。此法适用于树脂类、动物粪便类等容易相互粘结的药材。

辅料用量：一般为每100kg药物，用米醋20～30kg。

适用药物：具有峻下逐水作用的药物，如芫花；具有疏肝理气作用的药物，如柴胡；具有活血化瘀作用的药物，如延胡索；具有不良气味的药物，如乳香。

2. Stir-frying with Vinegar

Definition: Stir-frying with vinegar refers to the processing method that stir-fries purified or cut drugs with a certain amount of vinegar, and stir-fries them to a certain degree with low heat.

Purposes: ① Lead the effects of drugs to the liver meridian, to strengthen the effects of promoting blood circulation for removing blood stasis and regulating qi to alleviate pain. For example, the main effect of Bupleuri Radix (Chaihu) stir-fried with vinegar is to relieve stagnation of qi of liver. The main effect of Corydalis Rhizoma (Yanhusuo) stir-fried with vinegar is to promote blood circulation for removing blood stasis and stop the pain. ② Reduce drugs' toxicity and side-effects. For example, the main effect of Genkwa Flos (Yuanhua) stir-fried with vinegar is to remove water retention by strong diarrhea. ③ Rectify drugs' taste and smell. For example, the main effect of Olibanum (Ruxiang) stir-fried with vinegar is to modify its bad odor. ④ Make drugs easy to be crushed and decocted to get more effective components. For example, the texture of the mineral (Pyritum - Zirantong) and the shellfish (Testudinis Carapax et Plastrum- Guijia) would be transformed from hard to crisp after being processed.

Technics: There are two kinds of processing technologies.

Mix vinegar with drugs firstly and then fry. The operation is as follows: mix the purified or cut drugs with vinegar evenly, moisten them, but the drugs into a frying container, after the vinegar is absorbed thoroughly, fry them with mild fire to some certain degree, and take them out to become cool. The method is suitable for most drugs.

Fry drugs firstly and then sprinkle vinegar on the drugs' surface. Put the purified drugs into a frying container, then fry them to some certain degree, then sprinkle vinegar evenly on the drugs' surfaces, fry them slightly dry, take the drugs out of the container, turn them over and over again, and spread out to become cool. This way is suitable for those drugs which are easy to stick together after being processed.

Amount of adjuvant material: The amount of adjuvant material should be 20~30kg vinegar per 100kg drug.

Suitable drugs for application: This processing method is suitable for those drugs with the effect of drastic hydragogue (Genkwa Flos-Yuanhua), drugs with the effect of soothing liver and regulating qi (Bupleuri Radix-Chaihu), blood–activating and stasi–resolving drug (Corydalis Rhizoma-Yanhusuo), and drugs with bad odor (Olibanum-Ruxiang).

3. 盐炙法

定义：将净选或切制后的药物，加入一定量食盐水溶液用文火拌炒的方法。

目的：①盐炙能引药入肾。例如，杜仲的主要功效为补肝肾，强筋骨。盐炙后可引药入肾经并增强其功效。②盐炙可增强药效。例如，黄柏的主要作用为泻火解毒，清热燥湿。经过盐炙之后，可缓和苦燥之性，并可引药入肾经以泻肾火。③缓和药性。例如，盐炙可以缓和补骨脂的辛燥之性。

工艺：①先拌盐水后炒。适用于大多数药物。将药物与食盐水混合均匀，放置闷润，置于炒制容器内，用文火炒至盐水被吸尽，取出晾凉。②先炒药后加盐水。适用于含黏液质较多的药物，如车前子。先将药物置于炒制容器内，用文火炒至一定程度，再喷淋盐水，炒干，取出晾凉。

辅料用量：通常每 100kg 药物，用食盐 2kg，水 8～10kg。

适用药物：多用于补肾固精、疗疝、利尿和泻相火的药物。

3. Stir-frying with saltwater

Definition: Stir-frying with salt solution refers to the processing method that mixes a certain amount of salt solution with purified or cut drugs and stir-fries them with mild fire.

Purposes: ① The processing method helps to conduct the effects of drugs on the kidney meridian. For example, the main effects of the raw drugs of Eucommiae Cortex (Duzhong) are to replenish the liver and kidney, to strengthen muscle and bone, and to prevent abortion. After being processed with salt solution, the effects of the drug would be conducted on kidney meridian and would be strengthened. ② Stir-frying with the salt solution could enhance drugs' effects. For example, the main effects of raw products of Phellodendri Chinensis Cortex (Huangbai) are to purge pathogenic fire, detoxicate, and clear heat and dry dampness. After being stir-fried with salt solution, the bitter taste and dryness of the raw drug would be moderated. The effects could be conducted on kidney meridian to purge away pathogenic fire in the kidney. ③ Moderate drugs' nature. For example, the pungent and dry nature of Fructus Psoraleae (Buguzhi) would be moderated after being processed with sail solution.

Technics: There are two kinds of processing technologies. ① Mix drugs with a salt solution first then fry. It is suitable for most drugs. Mix the drugs with salt solution evenly, moisten them thoroughly, put them into a frying container, then fry them with mild fire until the salt solution is absorbed completely, then take the drugs out of the container to make them cool. ② fry drugs first and then sprinkle salt solution on the drugs' surface. it is suitable for those drugs with phlegmatic temperament (such as Semen Plantaginis - Cheqianzi). Put drugs into a frying container and fry with mild fire to a certain degree, then sprinkle salt solution evenly on the drugs' surface and fry them until they become. Finally, take the drugs out and make them cool.

Amount of adjuvant material: The amount of adjuvant material should be 2kg salt with 8kg~10kg water per 100kg drug.

Suitable drugs for application: This method is suitable for those drugs with the effect of invigorating kidney and astringing fluid, treating hernia, promoting diuresis, and purging the kidney heat.

4. 姜炙法

定义：将净选或切制后的药物，加入定量姜汁用文火加热拌炒至一定程度的方法。

目的：①缓和药性。例如，黄连姜炙可制其过于苦寒之性，使药性缓和。②增强和胃止呕作用。例如，黄连经过姜炙之后可增强止呕作用，砂仁经过姜炙可增强温胃止呕的功效，而竹茹姜炙长于降逆止呕。③减少刺激性。例如，厚朴对咽喉有一定的刺激性，姜炙可缓和其刺激性，并能增强温中化湿除胀的功效；半夏生品具有刺激性，经过姜炙之后，刺激性降低，并能增强其降逆止呕的作用。

工艺：①先加辅料后炒，此方法从新鲜生姜榨取或研磨得到姜汁。将药物与一定量的姜汁拌匀，放置闷润，使姜汁逐渐深入药物内部。置于炒制容器内，用文火炒至一定程度，取出晾凉。②姜汤煮，将鲜姜片煎汤，加入药物煮两小时，待姜汁基本被吸尽，取出，进行干燥，切片。

辅料用量：每100kg药物，用生姜10kg或干姜0.3kg。

适用药物：多用于祛痰止咳、降逆止呕的药物。

4. Stir-frying with ginger juice

Definition: Stir-frying with ginger juice refers to the processing method that to mix a certain amount of ginger juice with the purified or cut drugs and stir – fry them with mild fire to some degree.

Purposes: ① Moderate drugs' nature. For example, the nature of raw products of Goptidis Rhizoma (Huanglian) is bitter and cold, after being processed with ginger juice, nature could be moderated. ② Strengthen the drugs' effect of regulating stomachs for stopping vomiting. For example, after being processed with ginger juice, Goptidis Rhizoma (Huanglian) could stop vomiting, Fructus Amomi (Sharen) could warm stomachs to stop vomiting, and Bambusae Caulis in Taenia (Zhuru) could calm adverse – rising energy to stop vomiting. ③ Reduce drugs' irritation. For example, the main effect of the raw products of Magnoliae Officinalis Cortex (Houpo) is likely to stimulate throats. After being stir-fried with ginger juice, the irritation could be reduced; the effects of warning middle – energizer, resolving dampness, and relieving stagnation of qi could be strengthened. The raw products of Rhizoma Pinelliae Rhizoma (Banxia) have irritation and astringency, after being stir-fried with ginger juice, the irritation could be reduced, the effect of calming adverse – rising energy to stop vomiting would be strengthened.

Technics: There are two kinds of processing technologies. ① Mix ginger juice with drugs first and then fry. Ginger juice could be got by grinding fresh ginger or decocting Zingiberis rhizome. To be specific, it is to put drugs and ginger juice together, mix them thoroughly and moisten them completely, make the ginger juice penetrate gradually into the inner parts of the drugs. Put the drugs into a frying container and fry with mild fire to some certain degree, and finally take the drugs out and make them cool. ② Boil drugs with ginger juice together. Firstly, boil the fresh ginger and some water together to get the ginger juice. Then, add the drugs into the juice and continue to boil for four hours. When the ginger juice is almost absorbed by the drugs, take out the drugs, dry them, and cut them into slices.

Amount of adjuvant material: The amount of adjuvant material needed in the processing should be 10kg fresh ginger or 10/3 kg Zingiberis Rhizoma per 100kg drugs.

Suitable drugs for application: This processing method is suitable for those drugs with the effects of stopping coughing and eliminating phlegm and checking the adverse rise of qi to stop vomiting.

5. 蜜炙法

定义：将净选或切制后的药物，加入一定量炼蜜用文火拌炒至一定程度的方法。蜜炙法所使用的蜂蜜都要先加热炼过。

目的：①增加药物有效性。如百部蜜炙后能增强润肺止咳的作用；黄芪原药材的主要作用是益气固表，蜜炙能起到协同作用，增强其补中益气的功效。②缓和药性。例如，马兜铃生品味苦、性寒，具有清肺降气、止咳平喘的功能，经过蜜炙之后，能缓和其药性，并增强润肺止咳的功效；麻黄生品具有发汗解表的功效，经过蜜炙之后，缓和了辛散发汗的作用，以宣肺平喘力胜。③矫味和消除副作用。例如，马兜铃生品易致恶心呕吐，经过蜜炙之后，能矫正其不良气味，并减少呕吐的副作用。

工艺：①先拌蜜后炒药，适用于质地酥脆的药物。先取一定量的炼蜜，加适量开水稀释，与药物拌匀，放置闷润，使药物逐渐渗入药物组织内部，然后置于锅内，用文火炒至颜色加深、不黏手时，取出摊凉。②先炒药后加蜜，适用于质地致密的药物。先将药物置于锅内，用文火炒至颜色加深时，再加入一定量的炼蜜，迅速翻动，使蜜与药物拌匀，炒至不黏手，取出摊凉。

辅料用量：通常为每100kg药物，用炼蜜25kg。

注意事项：炼蜜若过于浓稠，可加适量开水稀释；炼蜜必须与药物充分拌匀闷润，使蜜完全渗入药物组织内部；蜜炙时，火力一定要小，以免焦化；蜜炙药物须凉后密闭贮存，并放置阴凉处，不宜受日光直接照射。

适用药物：多用于止咳平喘、补脾益气的药物。

5. Stir-frying with refined honey

Definition: Stir-frying with honey refers to the processing method that mixes refined honey into purified or cut drugs and stir-fries them with mild fire to some degree. In this method, the honey should be refined by heating before using in processing.

Purposes: ① Honey has synergistic action and could enhance drugs' effectiveness. For example, the main effect of the raw product of Stemonae Radix (Baibu) is to stop coughing and eliminate phlegm. After they are stir-fried with honey, the effect of moistening the lung and stopping cough would be strengthened. The main effect of the raw product of Astragali Radix (Huangqi) is to tonify qi and strengthen the exterior. After they are stir-fried with honey, the synergistic action of honey could strengthen the effect of tonifying the middle energizer and invigorating qi. ② Honey helps to moderate drugs' nature. For example, the raw product of Aristolochiae Fructus (Madouling) is bitter in flavor and cold in nature and has the effects of clearing the heat of the lung and depressing qi, and relieving cough and asthma. After it is stir-fried with honey, nature could be moderated, and the effect of moistening the lung and stopping coughing could be strengthened. The raw product of Ephedrae Herba (Mahuang) has the functions of inducing sweating and dispelling exogenous evils. After they are stir-fried with honey, the pungent dispersing and perspiration effect could be moderated. The main effect is to disperse lung qi to stop asthma. ③ Honey helps to modify the drugs' taste and eliminate the side effects. For example, the raw product of Aristolochiae Fructus (Madouling) is easy to cause and vomiting, after they are stir-fried with honey, the bad taste could be moderated and the side effect of vomiting could be eliminated.

Technics: There are two kinds of processing technologies. ① Mix honey with drugs first and then fry. It is suitable for drugs with a crisp texture. Dilute some refined honey with a certain amount of boiled water, then put into the honey, mix thoroughly and moisten thoroughly, and make the honey penetrate the inner part of the drugs; put the drugs into a preheating pan and fry with mild fire until the drugs show a deep color and with no sticking. Finally, take the drugs out of the pan and spread them to make them cool. ② Fry drugs first and then sprinkle honey on the drugs' surface. It is suitable for those drugs of dense texture.

Put drugs into a preheating pan and fry with mild fire, when the drugs become deep in color, pour some refined honey evenly on the drugs' surface and fry quickly, mix them thoroughly; when there is no sticking, take the drugs out of the pan and spread them to make them cool.

Amount of adjuvant material: The amount of adjuvant material needed in the processing is normally 25kg honey per 100kg drug.

Notices: The refined honey should be diluted with boiled water to make it not so vicious. The drugs and the refined honey should be mixed fully and moistened thoroughly. This is to make sure that honey could penetrate the inner parts of the drugs. During the process, the power should be mild so as not to parch the drugs. The drugs processed with honey should be stored and placed at cool places, avoiding sunlight and with the container closed tightly.

Suitable drugs for application: This method is suitable for the drugs with effects of relieving cough and asthma and invigorating middle energizer and tonifying qi.

6. 油炙法

定义：将净选或切制后的药物，与一定量的食用油脂共同加热处理的方法。

目的：增强药物温肾助阳的作用；利于粉碎，便于制剂和服用。

工艺：①油炒。取药物与油充分拌匀，置于炒制容器内，用文火快速炒至油被吸尽。每100kg药物，用油20kg。②油炸。将油倒入锅内加热，至沸腾时，倾入药物，用文火炸至药物酥脆为度。每100kg药物，用油25kg。③油烤。药物切成块放炉火上烤热，用油涂布，加热烘烤，待油渗入药内后，再涂再烤，反复操作，直至药物质地酥脆。

五、煅法

【定义】将药物直接或间接用火煅烧，使质地松脆或改变药物的理化性质。

【分类】煅法分为明煅法、煅淬法、暗煅法。

【注意事项】煅制药物时，要达到煅至"存性"的质量要求。例如，用闷煅法煅制一些植物类药材。药物必须大小分档，以免煅制时生熟不均。临床应用时，药物必须磨成粉末。

【适用药物】煅法主要适用于矿物类中药，以及质地坚硬的贝壳类、化石类药物。煅淬法适用于质地坚硬的矿物药，以及临床上因特殊需要而必须煅淬的药物。闷煅法适用于炒炭易灰化的制炭药物。

1. 明煅法

定义：直火煅法。

目的：①增强药效。例如，钟乳石经明煅后温肾壮阳作用增强。②改变药物的性质和药效。例如，生石膏具有清热泻火、除烦止渴的功效，经明煅后的煅石膏则具有收湿、敛疮、止血的功能。③降低毒性。例如，花蕊石煅后能缓和酸涩之性，消除伤脾伐胃的作用；寒水石煅后降低大寒之性。

6. Stir-frying with oil

Definition: Stir-frying with oil refers to the processing method that co – heats purified or cut drugs with a certain amount of oil.

Purposes: Strengthen drugs' effect of warming kidney to invigorate yang.

Make drugs easy to be crushed, facilitate preparation and taking.

Technics: There are three kinds of processing technologies.

Stir-frying with oil. Mix drugs with oil evenly put them into a frying container, fry them quickly with mild fire until the oil is absorbed thoroughly by the drugs. 20kg oil per 100kg drugs.

Frying drugs in oil. Heat oil in a pot until it boils, then pour the drugs in and fry them deeply with mild fire until the drugs become crisp. 25kg oil per 100kg drugs.

Baking drugs with oil. Cut drugs into clumps, bake them on fire, coat the drugs with oil and bake until the oil penetrates the inner parts of the drugs. Repeat the coating and baking procedure until the drugs become crisp.

Section Five　Calcining Method

【 **Definition** 】 The method of calcining drugs with direct fire.

【 **Classification** 】 Three types of methods include calcining openly, calcining and quenching, and hermetic calcining.

【 **Notices** 】 Drugs' inherent nature should be kept after being calcined. For example, the method of hermetic calcining can be used in processing some plant drugs to avoid being ashed. Drugs should be separated by size to avoid unevenness in the processing degree. Drugs should be ground into powders for clinical applications.

【 **Suitable drugs for application** 】 The method of calcining with direct fire is suitable for drugs of minerals, shellfish, and fossils. The calcining and quenching method is suitable for mineral drugs with harder texture or drugs for special needs in clinical applications, the method of hermetic calcining is suitable for drugs that are easy to be ashed in charring.

1. Calcining with Direct Fire

Definition: It means calcining with direct fire.

Purposes: ① Strengthen effects. For example, after being calcined, the effect of warming the kidney to invigorate yang of Stalactitum (Zhongrushi) would be strengthened. ② Change drugs' nature and effects. For example, the main effects of raw product of Gypsum Fibrosum (Shigao) are to clear heat and purge away pathogenic fire, relieve restlessness and thirst. After being calcined, the main effects of dried Gypsum are to arrest dampness and ulceration to stop bleeding. ③ Reduce toxicity. For example, after being calcined, the main effects of Ophicalcitum (Huaruishi) are to moderate acidity, impair the spleen and stomach. The great cold nature of Calcium (Hanshuishi) could also be moderated.

工艺：①直接煅法。将药物直接加热或煅烧，煅至红透后取出，临床使用时粉碎。②间接煅法，将药物置于耐火容器中再放入炉火中加热，煅至红透。临床使用时粉碎。

注意事项：煅至完全且煅制过程中不能搅拌；煅制温度、时间要适度；煅制过程中以防爆溅；药物彻底凉透后储存。

2. 煅淬法

定义：将药物按明煅法煅至红透后，立即投入规定的液体辅料中骤然冷却的方法称煅淬。常用的淬液有水、醋、酒或药汁。

目的：①使药物质地酥脆，易于粉碎，利于有效成分煎出。②改变药物的理化性质，减少副作用，增强疗效。③消除毒性、清除杂质。

工艺：将药物按明煅法煅至红透后取出，立即投入液体辅料中。反复多次直至药物质松易碎。

注意事项：许多药物煅淬要反复多次；煅淬时药物要吸尽醋、酒、药汁等淬液；根据各药物的性质和煅淬目的要求不通的淬液种类和用量。

3. 暗煅法

定义：药物在高温缺氧条件下煅烧成炭的方法。

目的：①产生或增强止血作用，如血余炭、棕榈炭。②降低毒性，如干漆、蜂房。

工艺：将药物置于锅中，再盖一较小的锅，两锅结合处用盐泥封严，盖锅上压一重物，用武火加热煅制成炭。

判断标准：滴水于盖锅底部即沸；盖锅底部贴张白纸，煅至纸呈深黄色即可；盖锅底部放几粒大米，煅至大米呈深黄色即可；两锅密封处裂隙冒出的烟雾由黑变白即可。

注意事项：煅炭防灰化；煅锅内药料放置适量，避免煅制不透；药物凉透后开锅。

Technics: ① Direct method. Put drugs in heater or fire, calcine thoroughly until the drugs become flaming red inside, and take them out of the container. Crush when used in the clinic. ② Indirect method. Put drugs in a refractory container, then put the container in a heater or over the fire, and calcine thoroughly until the drugs become flaming red inside. Crush when used in the clinic.

Notices: Calcine thoroughly without stirring. Choose a suitable time and temperature. Avoid exploding and spilling when calcining. Store after drugs being cool.

2. Calcining and quenching

Definition: After being calcined thoroughly the drugs are added into a quenching liquid as soon as possible to get drugs cool suddenly. The quenching liquids include water, vinegar, wine, or drugs' juice.

Purposes: ① Make drugs' texture crisper and easy to be crushed, which is good for decocting of the effective ingredients. ② Change drugs' physico – chemical properties, whiled reduce side – effects and strengthen drugs' effects. ③ Reduce toxicity and remove foreign materials.

Technics: Put drugs in a heater or over a fire, calcine thoroughly until the drugs become flaming red inside, and take drugs out of the container. Then put drugs into quenching liquid quickly. Repeat the procedure several times if needed until the drugs' texture becomes crisper.

Notices: Drugs processed by this method should be calcined and quenched repeatedly. If the quenching liquid is vinegar, wine, or drugs' juice, they should be absorbed thoroughly by drugs. Choose suitable quenching liquids according to the processing purpose and drugs' nature.

3. Hermetic calcining

Definition: It means calcining drugs to a carbonized state at a high temperature without oxygen.

Purposes: ① Produce or strengthen hemostasis effect, for example, Crinis Carbonisatus (Xueyutan), Petiolus Trachycarpi Carbonisatus (Zonglvtan). ② Reduce toxicity, for example, Toxicodendri Resina (Ganqi), Vespae Nidus (Fengfang).

Technics: Put drugs in a big pot with a small pot covered with weights. Be closed by brine sludge or sand and calcined with high temperature.

Standards: Water boils as soon as it drips on the bottom of the covered small pot. The paper on the bottom of the covered small pot transforms from white to yellow. The rice on the bottom of the covered small pot transforms from white to yellow. The color of smoke from the fissure transforms from black to white during processing.

Notices: Char but without ashing. During processing, suitable amounts should be used to avoid charring unevenly. Open the pot after drugs are thoroughly cool.

六、蒸煮燀法

蒸、煮、燀法为一类"水火共制"法。这里的"水"可以是清水,也可以是酒、醋或药汁。

1. 蒸法

定义:将净选或切制后的药物加辅料(酒、醋、药汁等)或不加辅料装入蒸制容器内隔水加热至一定程度的方法。直接利用流通蒸汽蒸者称为"直接蒸法";药物在密闭条件下隔水蒸者称"间接蒸法",又称"炖法"。

目的:①改变药性,扩大用药范围。如地黄生品性寒,清热凉血,蒸制后使药性转温,味道由苦转甜,功能由清变补。②减少副作用。如大黄酒蒸后苦寒作用缓和,并能减轻腹痛等副作用。③保存药效,利于储存。如桑螵蛸生品经蒸后杀死虫卵,便于储存。④便于软化切片。如黄芩不能在冷水中软化,以免有效成分损失,蒸后便于软化切片。

工艺:第一种方法是将药物加辅料或不加辅料放在蒸制容器内,用蒸汽加热蒸到一定程度的方法;第二种方法是将药物加液体辅料,如酒,放置在密闭容器内用蒸汽加热到一定程度的方法。

注意事项:须用液体辅料拌蒸的药物应待辅料被吸尽后再蒸制;加液体辅料蒸制时必须采取第二种方法;蒸制时一般先用武火,再用文火。

适用药物:主要适用于通过蒸制可以改变药物性味的药物,特别是滋阴补血的药物。

2. 煮法

定义:将净选过的药物加辅料或不加辅料放入锅内(固体辅料须先捣碎或切制),加适量清水同煮的方法。

Section Six Steaming, Boiling, and Blanching

The method of steaming, boiling, and blanching means preparing drugs with liquid and fire together. The "liquid" includes clean water, wine, vinegar, or drugs' juice.

1. Steaming method

Definition: It is a method that steams the drugs which are cut or purified with or without adjuvant materials (wine, vinegar, or drugs juice) to some degree. The method of steaming indirect vapor is called "direct steam". While steaming in a tightly closed container is called "indirect steam" or "Stewing".

Purposes: ① Change drugs' nature and enlarge clinical usage. For example, the nature of the raw Rehmanniae Radix (Dihuang) is cold. The effects are to remove heat and cool blood. After steaming, nature changes from coldness to warmness, from bitterness to sweetness. The main effect changes from clearing to nourishing. ② Reduce side – effects. For example, after steaming, the cold and bitter nature of Rhei Radix Et Rhizoma (Daihuang) could be moderated and the side effect of drastic purgation would be reduced. ③ Remain efficacy and be good for storing. For example, after steaming, the eggs of Mantidis Ootheca (Sangpiaoxiao) would be killed to store. ④ Facilitate softening of drugs. For example, Scutellariae Radix (Huangqin) should not be softened in cold water to avoid loss of effective components, it can be easily softened and cut after being steamed.

Technics: The first method is to put drugs with or without adjuvant materials in a steam container, steaming drugs to some degree.

The second method is to put drugs with liquid adjuvant materials, such as wine, in a closed container, steaming drugs to some degree.

Notices: The drugs steaming with liquid adjuvant materials should be steamed after the adjuvant materials being absorbed thoroughly. The second method should be adopted when steaming drugs with liquid adjuvant materials. The principle of steaming is "strong fire first and then mild fire". To avoid drying out, drugs need to be steamed for a long should keep adding hot water into the steam container.

Suitable drugs for application: It is suitable for those drugs whose nature would be changed by steaming, especially the drugs that can nourish yin and tonify blood.

2. Boiling method

Definition: It means boiling drugs with or without adjuvant materials (solid adjuvant materials should be pounded or cut to pieces before boiling) in water to some degree.

目的：①消除或降低药物的毒副作用。如川乌生品的毒性经煮制后明显降低；硫黄与豆腐同煮（每100kg净硫磺，用豆腐200kg）后，毒性降低，可增强助阳益火的作用。②改变药性，增强药效。如远志用甘草水煮减其燥性，协同增强安神益智的功效。③清洁药物。如珍珠经豆腐煮后可去其油腻，便于服用。

工艺：将药物加辅料或不加辅料放入锅内，加适量水，先用武火加热，煮沸后再用文火煮至一定程度。煮法可分为3种，清水煮、加辅料煮（先加辅料闷润后煮和先加辅料后投入药物共煮）、豆腐煮。

原则：武火煮至沸腾后，改用文火煎煮。

注意事项：煮制过程中及时补充水量；文火保持微沸；大小分档，分别炮制；煮好后出锅，及时烘干或晒干。

适用药物：适用于毒性药物或需增强药效的药物，如川乌、远志、珍珠。

3. 燀法

定义：将药物置于沸水中浸煮短暂时间，取出，分离种皮的方法。

目的：①增强药效，如桃仁。②分离不同的药用部位，如白扁豆。③降低毒性，如苦杏仁。

工艺：先将多量清水加热至沸腾，再把药物投入沸水中，稍微翻烫数分钟，立即取出，浸漂于冷水中，捞起，搓开种皮、种仁，再筛去种皮。

注意事项：水量一般为药量的10倍以上；药物要燀至种皮由皱缩到膨胀，易于挤脱时方可；燀制时间要短，一般为5～10分钟左右；燀制过程中，温度要高，以防止药物有效成分被酶解；燀去皮后，宜晒干或低温烘干。

Purposes: ① Remove or decrease toxicity and side effects. For example, the toxicity of the raw Aconiti Kusnezoffii Radix (Chuanwu) would be reduced after boiling. Boling Sulfer (Liuhuang) with bean curd (200kg bean curd per 100kg sulfur) would reduce the toxicity and enhance the effect of warning kidney to invigorate yang and dejection. ② Change drugs' nature and strengthen effects. For example, after boiling with Radix Glycyrrhizae juice, the dryness of Polygalae Radix (Yuanzhi) would be moderated and the effect of calming the nerves and reinforcing intelligence would be strengthened. ③ Clean drugs. For example, after boiling with bean curd, the grease of pearl would be removed and easy to use.

Technics: Put drugs and clear water together, with or without adjuvant materials, heat drugs with strong fire at first, and then keep boiling with mild fire to some degree. The methods of boiling can be divided into three types, which include boiling without adjuvant materials, boiling with adjuvant materials (Which can be divided into soaking in adjuvant materials first and then boiling, and decocting adjuvant materials first and then put drugs to boil together), and boiling with bean curd.

Principle: Heat with a strong fire at first and then keep boiling with mild fire.

Notices: Remember to add suitable water when boiling. Keep boiling with mild fire. Before boiling, drugs should be separated by size to keep processing evenly and thoroughly. Dry timely after finishing boiling.

Suitable drugs for application: It is suitable for toxic drugs or drugs which need to enhance effects, such as Polygalae Radix (Yuanzhi), Margarita (Zhenzhu).

3. Blanching method

Definition: It means heating drugs in boiling water for a short time to separate seed coat and kernel.

Purposes: ① Enhance effects. Take Persicae Semen (Taoren) for example. ② Separate different medicinal parts. Take Lablab Semen Album (Baibiandou) for example. ③ Reduce toxicity. Take Lablab Semen Album for example.

Technics: Boil plenty of clear water and put the drugs in. after several minutes, take them out immediately, and put into cold water as soon as possible, take them out, and knead to separate seed coat and kernel, screen out the coat.

Notices: The amount of water should be more than ten times the amount of drugs. Heat drugs till the outer part of the seed's coat changes from shrinking to expanding and easy to squeeze out the kernel. The time of blanching should be within a short time, normally 5 to 10 minutes. During blanching, keep a high temperature to prevent some effective components from being enzymolyzed. Dry under the sun or use oven drying with low temperature.

七、其他方法

1. 复制法

定义：用数种辅料反复炮制药物的方法。

目的：①减少或除去毒性成份。例如，生半夏所含成分是有毒的并具有刺激性，会致呕吐，所以常常外用。使用复制法炮制后，其毒性和刺激性有所减轻。②矫臭矫味。例如，紫河车用酒和花椒炮制后，除去了腥臭味。③改变药物性质，增强药物疗效，或者扩大临床应用。例如，生天南星所含成分的性味是辛温的，主要功效是消除寒痰。用胆汁炮制后，性由温转寒，主要功效是清除热痰。

工艺：将药物放入一种或数种辅料中，通过水浸或加热处理，直到药物达到规定的程度。

注意事项：此方法包含许多过程，因此花费时间较长，用到辅料较多。

适用药物：适用于有毒药物，如半夏、白附子、天南星。

2. 发酵发芽法

定义：借助酶的分解和腐化作用，使药物发芽和发酵，从而达到改变药物性质，增强和产生新的功效。

条件：①发酵条件包括酵母、微生物、适宜的温度和湿度。②发芽条件包括选种，适宜的温度、湿度和时间。发芽或发酵后，大部分药物要经过油煎处理。

（1）发酵法

定义：在适宜的温度和湿度下，利用霉菌催化分解，使药物发泡或纯化的方法。

作用：①产生新的疗效。例如，六神曲具有健脾和促进食欲的作用。建曲具有祛除风寒，健脾和胃。淡豆豉主要功效是解表除烦。②改变药物性质，增强药物疗效。例如，半夏发酵后成为半夏曲，主要功效为健脾暖胃，燥湿化痰。

Section Seven   Other Ways

1. Duplication method

Definition: It refers to processing drugs repeatedly with several adjuvant materials.

Purposes: ① Reduce or eliminate toxicity. For example, the ingredients of raw Rhizoma Pinelliae Rhizoma (Banxia) are toxic and irritant and can cause vomiting, so it is mostly used externally. After being processed by duplication methods, the toxicity and irritation could be moderated. ② Modify smell and taste. For example, the bad odor of Placenta Hominis (Ziheche) could be moderated by processing with wine and Pericarpium Zanthoxyli (Huajiao). ③ Change the nature of drugs, improve drug efficacy or expand the clinical application. For example, the nature of the products of raw Arisaematis Rhizoma (Tiannanxing) is pungent and warm, and its main function is removing cold phlegm. After being processed by bile, the warm nature becomes cold and the main function is to clear away heat phlegm.

Technics: Mix drugs with one or several adjuvant materials together, and process them by immersing in water or heating until the drugs get to the extent of regulation.

Notices: This method includes many procedures, so it often takes a long time and asks for many adjuvant materials.

Suitable drugs for application: Toxic drugs, such as Rhizoma Pinelliae Rhizoma (Banxia), Typhonii Rhizoma (Baifuzi), and Arisaematis Rhizoma (Tiannanxing).

2. Methods of Fermenting and Sprouting

Definition: It changes the nature of drugs strengthens drug efficacy and produces new functions through fermenting and sprouting with catalysis and decomposition of enzyme.

Condition: ① Fermenting condition: yeast, microbes, suitable temperature, and dampness are needed. ② Sprouting condition: seed selection, suitable temperature, dampness and time are necessary. After fermenting or sprouting, most drugs need to be further processed.

(1) Fermenting

Definition: It refers to the method that makes drugs ferment or is purified with catalysis and decomposition of mold under suitable temperature and dampness.

Functions: ① Produce new functions. For example, after being processed, the main effects of Massa Medicata Fermentata (Liushenqu) are invigorating spleens and improving appetite. The main effects of Medicinal Fermented Mass are promoting digestion, expelling wind-cold, invigorating spleens, and regulating stomachs. The main effects of Sojae Semen Preparatum (Dandouchi) are relieving superficies and eliminating irritability. ② Change the nature of drugs and enhance drug efficacy. For example, after being processed, the main effects of Rhizoma Pinelliae Rhizomae (Banxia) fermented mass are invigorating spleens, warming stomachs, and drying dampness to resolve phlegm.

专属条件：发酵的适宜温度是 30～37℃，相对湿度是 70%～80%，其他条件还包括培养基，pH 值 4～7.6，足够的氧气或者二氧化碳。

判断标准：成品表面黄白色，内部有斑点，同时带有酵香气，不应出现黑色及酸败味。

注意事项：药物在发酵前，要先进行杀虫、杀菌处理；发酵过程不能中断；发酵过程要时刻注意温度和湿度。

（2）发芽法

定义：在适宜温度和湿度条件下，使药物提纯或发芽的方法。

作用：经过萌芽，淀粉可以被分解为糊精、葡萄糖及果糖，蛋白质可以被分解为氨基酸，脂肪可以分解为甘油和脂肪酸。同时，会产生消化酶和维生素。所有这些变化将使药物产生新的效果。例如，经过发芽，麦芽具有促进消化、和胃、回奶的作用。

专属条件：在发芽前，应通过发芽能力测试，应达 85% 以上，芽的长度为 0.2～1cm。发芽适宜温度为 18～25℃，必须有足够的氧气。

工艺：在合适的温度和湿度下，将药物浸在水中直到发芽，干燥，得到成品。

3. 制霜法

定义：透过除油、提取、蒸发和煎煮法制得粉渣的方法。

注意事项：种子应该用加热和挤压方法进行去油，矿物质制霜最好在秋天进行。

适用药物：种子、矿物质、动物的角。

（1）去油制霜法

目的：降低毒性，缓和药性，降低副作用。例如，巴豆经去油制霜后，其峻猛的泻下作用得到缓和。

工艺：除去药物的外壳，取得内核，将药物研细，用纸或布包裹。蒸后，将药物放在阳光下晒干，榨去油，如此重复数次，直到药物松散成粉。

注意事项：药物经过处理后，所用的纸或布应该尽快丢弃，以避免中毒；在处理过程中，必须进行加热；巴豆霜的油脂含量应为 18%～20%。

Special condition: The suitable temperature and relative dampness for fermenting are 30~37℃ and 70%~80% respectively. Other conditions include culture medium, pH4~7.6, and enough oxygen or carbon dioxide.

Standards: The processed products should be yellowish-white on their surfaces, spots inside, and the fermented smell comes out. The black color and rancidity – odor should be avoided.

Notices: Preprocess with anthelminthic and disinfection before fermenting is necessary. No interrupting during the process of fermentation. Pay attention to the temperature and humidity all the time during fermentation.

(2) Sprouting

Definition: It refers to the method that makes drugs sprout or is purified under suitable temperature and dampness.

Condition: After sprouting, starch in drugs can be decomposed into artificial gum, glucose, and fructose; protein can be decomposed into amino acids; fats can be decomposed to glycerin and fatty acids, meanwhile, digestive enzymes and vitamins will be produced. All these changes will make drugs produce new effects. For example, after sprouting, malt has the functions of promoting digestion, regulating stomach, and delectation.

Special condition: Before being chosen to sprout, the seeds should be given germination capacity tests. The germination capacity should be more than 85%. The standard sprout length is 0.2 cm. During sprouting, the suitable temperature is 18~25℃. Enough oxygen is necessary.

Technics: Soak drugs in water under suitable temperature and dampness until they sprout, then dry them and get finished products.

3. Method of making frostlike powder

Definition: It means making frostlike powder through degreasing, extracting, evaporating, or decocting.

Notices: The method of heating and squeezing should be used for seeds' degreasing. Minerals should be processed on cool autumn days.

Suitable drugs for application: Seeds, minerals, and animal horns.

(1) Making frostlike powder with degreasing

Purposes: Reduce toxicity, moderate the nature of drugs and eliminate side effects. For example, the drastic purgation would be moderated after Fructus Crotonis (Badou) is defatted to powder.

Technics: Remove drugs' shell and get kernels, grind drugs into small pieces and wrap them with paper or cloth. After steaming, dry drugs in the sunshine, squeeze and discard the paper or cloth, then repeat the procedure several times till getting frostlike powder.

Notices: After being processed, the paper or cloth should be discarded as soon as possible to avoid intoxication. During processing, heating is necessary. Content of grease should be 18%~20% in defatted croton seed powder.

（2）渗析制霜法

目的：制造新药，增加药物疗效。

（3）升华制霜法

目的：纯净药物。

工艺：将药物放在一大锅中，上面扣一小锅，小锅上加重物，结合处用盐泥或砂土封固，高温煅烧，收集盖锅上的升华结晶。

（4）煎煮制霜法

目的：缓和药性，扩大临床应用，扩大药源。

4. 烘焙法

定义：将净选或切制后的药物用文火直接或间接烘干的方法。

目的：使药物便于贮存，避免发霉；使药物易于粉碎；降低药物毒性。

工艺：一般的药物用烘箱或者干燥箱进行烘焙，动物类药物要用直火进行烘焙，在炮制过程中，用文火，并要不断地翻动药物。

5. 煨法

定义：将药物用湿纸或湿面粉包裹，放到加热的蛤粉或麦麸中，除去部分油脂的方法。

目的：减少副作用，缓和药效，增强疗效。

分类：煨法可以分为麦麸煨、面粉煨、滑石粉煨、纸或湿纸煨。

注意事项：在煨法中，要注意辅料煨和辅料炒之间的不同。例如，麦麸炒和麦麸煨，所需辅料量，在麦麸煨中，每100kg药材，用麦麸40kg；而在麦麸炒中，每100kg药材，用麦麸10～15kg。所用的火候，麦麸煨法中要用文火，炮制时间相对较长；麦麸炒法中用中火，炮制时间短。在操作步骤方面，麦麸煨法是将药物和麦麸同时放到锅里，麦麸炒法是先加热麦麸，再投入药物。

(2) Making frostlike powder with educing

Purposes: Make new drugs and improve drugs' efficacy.

(3) Making Frostlike Powder with Sublimating

Purposes: Purify drugs.

Technics: Put drugs in a big pot, and cover them with a small pot with heavy objects on. Seal the two pots with brine sludge or sand, calcined the drugs at high temperatures, then collect the crystals that sublimate on the bottom of the small pot.

(4) Method of making frostlike powder with decocting

Purposes: Moderate the nature of drugs, expand the clinical application and medicinal resources.

4. Methods of roasting or baking

Definition: It refers to the method that bakes purified or cut drugs with direct or indirect slow fire.

Purposes: Make drugs easy to be stored and avoid mold. Make drugs easy to be crushed. Reduce toxicity of drugs.

Technics: Most drugs are roasted in a baking oven or drying oven, while animal drugs are baked with direct fire. During processing, the heat level should be low and drugs need to be overturned continuously.

5. Method of roast in fresh cinders

Definition: It refers to the method that wraps drugs with wet paper or flour, and puts them in heated clam powders or bran to remove some grease.

Purposes: Reduce the side – effects of drugs, moderate their medical nature, and enhance their efficacy.

Classification: Roasting methods include roasting with bran, flour, talcum powder, paper, or wet paper.

Notices: During roasting, we should pay attention to the differences between roasting and stir-frying with adjuvant materials. Take roasting with bran and stir-frying with bran for example, for the dosage of adjuvant materials, the former ratio is 100:40, and the latter si 100:10~100:15. For the firepower and time, the former should be processed with a low fire and last for a relatively long time, and the latter should be processed with medium fire for less time. The operation procedure: the former asks for putting drugs and bran in a container together at the same time, and the latter asks for heating bran first and then adding drugs in a container.

6. 提净法

定义：通过溶解、过滤、重结晶的方法提纯一些矿物质类药物，特别是含有不容的无机盐的矿物质类药物。

目的：纯化药物，增加疗效；改变药物性质；减低毒性。

工艺：①降温结晶（冷结晶）。将药物与辅料共煮后，过滤，将滤液置阴凉处，使之冷却，收集结晶。②蒸发结晶（热结晶）。将药物与水共热直到药物溶解，过滤，收集滤液，在滤液中加醋混合，把水分蒸干，在滤液便面有结晶生成，收集结晶。

7. 水飞法

定义：利用粗细粉的不同性质，将不溶于水的药物与水反复研磨，分离得到细粉的方法。

目的：除去杂质，洁净药物；使药物质地细腻；在研磨过程中防止尘粉飞扬；降低毒性。

工艺：将药物与水研磨数分钟，再加水，使悬浮，倒出悬浮液，剩余部分再进行研磨，如此反复操作，使收集悬浮液静置，去掉上面的水，收集沉淀。

注意事项：在研磨时，水量应少；搅拌时水量宜大；晾干，不宜加热；研磨朱砂和雄黄时要忌铁器。

适用药物：适用于不溶于水的药物，如雄黄、朱砂、珍珠。

8. 干馏法

定义：将药物置于容器中焙烤使其产生干馏物的方法。

目的：制备有别于原药材的干馏物，以适合临床需要。

工艺：①上部收集液。收集冷凝液，例如，黑豆馏油就是用这种方法收集。②下部收集液。收集液体，例如，竹沥油就是用这种方法收集。③炒制收集物。收集油类物质，例如蛋黄油。

6. Method of defecating

Definition: It means purifying some minerals, especially soluble inorganic salt minerals through the procedure of dissolving, filtering, and recrystallization.

Purposes: Purify drugs and enhance efficacy. Alter the nature of drugs. Reduce the toxicity of drugs.

Technics: ① Lower the temperature for crystallizing (cold crystallizing). Boil drugs and adjuvant materials together, then filter them. Put the filtrate in a shady and cool place to make them cool, collect the crystals. ② Evaporate for crystallizing (hot crystallizing). Heat drugs and water together until drugs dissolve, filter and collect the filtrate, mix vinegar with the filtrate until the water evaporated. Then the crystals are reduced to the surface of the filtrate, collect the crystals.

7. Section seven grinding drugs in water

Definition: It refers to preparing fine powder of drugs which are insoluble in water through grinding drugs in water repeatedly according to different floating property of coarse and fine powder.

Purposes: Remove impurities and clean drugs. Make drugs exquisite. Avoid dust flying up during grinding. Reduce toxicity.

Technics: Grinding drugs with water for several minutes, add more water in and get the suspension, and pour out the suspension into another container. The remainder will be processed in the same way several times. Suspension is collected and kept still for some time. Then the precipitate is collected and the supernatant is discarded.

Notices: Less water during grinding. More water during stirring to get the suspension. Open-air drying and avoid heating. Avoid iron when grinding cinnabar and realgar.

Suitable drugs for application: It is suitable for drugs being insoluble in water, such as realgar, cinnabar, and pearl.

8. Method of dry distillation

Definition: It refers to baking or burning drugs in a container to produce pyrolysate.

Purposes: Produce new pyrolysate that is different from original drugs for clinical use.

Technics: ① Collect from the upper part, that is to collect condensate. For example, Pityrolum (Heidouliuyou) would be collected by this method. ② Collect from the lower part, that is to collect liquid from drugs directly. For example, juice of bamboo. Succus Bambusae would be collected by this method. ③ Collect by stir-frying, that is to collect the oily materials. For example, egg oil would be collected by this method.

参考文献：

[1] 刘振丽，宋志前，李淑莉.何首乌净选加工、切制和干燥方法对化学成分的影响[J].中草药，2004（04）：48-50.

[2] 汪海峰，杨杰.中药炮制去除非药用部位的意义探讨[J].西南军医，2015，17（06）：666-668.

[3] 傅宝庆.中药炮制中的"净选加工"对疗效的影响[J].中成药研究，1982（11）：19-20.

[4] 王素霞，徐亚民.中药饮片炮制前不同筛选方式对疗效的影响研究[J].中药与临床，2020，11（02）：16-18.

[5] 郑文杰，王振国.《本草纲目》中毒性药物的炮制[J].时珍国医国药，2018，29（08）：2007-2009.

[6] 王家骅，任玉基.中药去皮壳的合理性探讨[J].基层中药杂志，1992（01）：12-13.

[7] 代涛，李光燕，徐茂红.知母炮制方法的历史沿革与现代研究[J].中成药，2020，42（12）：3255-3258.

［8］尹子丽，谭文红，冯德强，等.骨碎补的本草考证及炮制、药用历史沿革［J］.中国药房，2019，30（12）：1725-1728.

［9］徐钢，鞠成国，于海涛，等.中药狗脊炮制研究进展［J］.中国实验方剂学杂志，2012，18（05）：238-242.

［10］高慧，黄雯，熊之琦，等.远志的炮制研究进展［J］.中国实验方剂学杂志，2020，26（23）：209-218.

［11］景海漪，史辑，贾天柱.巴戟天的炮制历史沿革［J］.中国药房，2013，24（27）：2575-2577.

［12］赫炎，王祝举，唐力英.牡丹皮炮制历史沿革研究［J］.中国实验方剂学杂志，2007（11）：67-68.

［13］李玉丽，蒋屏，杨恬，等.地骨皮的本草考证［J］.中国实验方剂学杂志，2020，26（05）：192-201.

［14］修彦凤，王兴发，吴弢，等.瓜蒌子的炮制历史沿革［J］.中草药，2003（12）：103-105.

［15］李玉丽，蒋屏，杨恬，等.地骨皮的本草考证［J］.中国实验方剂学

杂志，2020，26（05）：192-201.

[16]丁蓉.金樱子去核毛炮制体会[J].中国误诊学杂志，2011，11（07）：1630.

[17]曹岗，邵玉蓝，张云，等.山茱萸炮制历史沿革及现代研究[J].中草药，2009，40（S1）：69-71.

[18]乔立新.山楂去核问题的探讨[J].中国药房，2002（05）：56.

[19]孙红祥.诃子炮制历史沿革研究[J].中药材，1991（05）：31-33.

[20]祝婧，叶喜德，吴江峰，等.枳壳炮制历史沿革及炮制品现代研究进展[J].中国实验方剂学杂志，2019，25（20）：191-199.

[21]朱春晓，谢明，李昶，等.乌梢蛇的本草考证研究[J].中国现代中药，2018，20（12）：1573-1578.

[22]赵永德，张金凤.谈中药炮制中的"去"[J].滨州医学院学报，1990（03）：70-71.

[23]闫珍珲，李小芳，宋佳文，等.中药材的净制与切制研究进展[J].中药与临床，2019，10（02）：51-54.

[24] 周劲松, 张洪坤, 黄玉瑶, 等. 天麻不同软化方法的比较及天麻片炮制工艺优化研究 [J]. 时珍国医国药, 2016, 27 (03): 622-624.

[25] 修彦凤, 曹艳花, 王平. 多指标综合评价优选木瓜润法和蒸法软化的炮制工艺 [J]. 时珍国医国药, 2009, 20 (05): 1247-1249.

[26] 孙立立, 庄立品, 王琦, 等. 中药槟榔饮片切制工艺研究 [J]. 中成药, 1997 (11): 20-22.

[27] 杨俊杰, 张振凌. 中药饮片与其加工设备沿革的探讨 [J]. 时珍国医国药, 2010, 21 (04): 925-926.

[28] 葛迪. 不同炮制加工方法对桔梗饮片质量的影响 [J]. 西部中医药, 2019, 32 (05): 20-22.

[29] 肖国鑫, 朱琳, 周亮, 等. 真空冷冻干燥炮制法对藏天麻活性成分提取的影响 [J]. 经济林研究, 2016, 34 (01): 164-167.

[30] 陈璇. 不同干燥方法对玄参品质的影响 [D]. 武汉: 湖北中医药大学, 2010.

[31] 朱诗慧. 中药饮片质价关联的形成机制研究 [D]. 南京: 南京中医药

大学，2015.

［32］钟喜光，刘瑞连，蒋晓煌，等.揉搓对玉竹中多糖提取率影响的研究［J］.中国药物经济学，2013（S1）：208-209.

［33］韩俊生.中药"拌衣"炮制法的沿革与评价［J］.上海中医药杂志，2002（12）：38-39.

［34］杨培民，邵晓慧，刘咏梅.麻黄绒炮制研究［J］.中药材，1998（11）：564-565.

［35］燕娜娜，李丹，魏敏，等.不同火力炒制对白术成分含量的影响［J］.中药材，2020，43（02）：323-327.

［36］徐瑶."焦三仙"炒焦增强消食导滞的"焦香气味"物质及其协同增效作用机理研究［D］.成都：西南交通大学，2018.

［37］张韵.山楂炒焦机理及其焦香气味物质基础研究［D］.成都：西南交通大学，2016.

［38］陈缤，王丽娜，贾天柱.单炒的历史沿革研究［J］.中成药，2014，36（06）：1281-1284.

［39］钟凌云，龚千锋，张的凤.中药炒炭的炮制机理［J］.时珍国医国药，2002（01）：19.

［40］吴茂富，苗西成.炒黄、炒焦、炒炭的炮制分析［J］.黑龙江中医药，2000（01）：59-60.

［41］马嘉擎，赵小雨，刘艳艳，等.麸炒中药现代研究进展［J］.广东药科大学学报，2021，37（02）：163-166.

［42］王梅，荆然，王越欣，等.米炒党参的历史沿革及其现代炮制工艺、化学成分和药理作用的研究进展［J］.中国药房，2020，31（14）：1788-1792.

［43］黄清杰，徐志伟.砂炒法的历史沿革与研究进展［J］.甘肃医药，2020，39（04）：301-303.

［44］李楠，谭裕君，王念明，等.滑石粉炒鱼鳔胶炮制工艺优选［J］.中国药业，2017，26（13）：5-8.

［45］刘玉杰.砂炒马钱子炮制工艺优化与质量评价研究［D］.成都：成都中医药大学，2014.

［46］陈康林，陈鸿平，陈林.中药土炒炮制的历史沿革与现代研究进展

[J]．中外医疗，2009，28（01）：154-156．

［47］崔金玉．阿胶炮制工艺及质量控制研究［D］．沈阳：辽宁中医药大学，2008．

［48］徐凤娟，孙娥，张振海，等．中药炮制辅料羊脂油的研究思路探析[J]．中华中医药杂志，2014，29（08）：2543-2547．

［49］贺亚男，刘昱，王芳，等，杨明．杜仲炮制历史沿革及近20年研究进展［J］．中国现代中药，2021，23（4）：593-598．

［50］杨洁．浅谈姜制法与姜的药对配伍［J］．西部中医药，2013，26（04）：12-13．

［51］荣杰，张军平．盐炙法在中药炮制中的药效学研究［J］．时珍国医国药，2011，22（07）：1692-1693．

［52］李华鹏，桑立红，侯准，等．中药酒制的研究概况［J］．中药材，2011，34（03）：478-481．

［53］张泰，王学美．中药蜜制法沿革述要［J］．环球中医药，2009，2（03）：

220-222.

［54］王静，毛春芹，陆兔林.中药醋制法研究进展［J］.中国中医药信息杂志，2009，16（01）：99-101.

［55］李艳凤，翟梦颖，李雨昕，等.发酵法在中药研究中的应用［J］.医学综述，2020，26（04）：753-757.

［56］崔美娜，钟凌云，张大永，等.中药半夏复制法炮制的研究进展［J］.中国中药杂志，2020，45（06）：1304-1310.

［57］靳庆霞.朱砂水飞法炮制前后可溶性硫和汞的含量分析［J］.中国合理用药探索，2017，14（03）：12-14.

［58］陈晓红.浅谈中药炮制的煅法及其临床作用［J］.湖北中医学院学报，2009，11（06）：39-40.

［59］冯建华，陈秀琼.中药炮制"煨法"考证［J］.时珍国医国药，2004，15（06）：338-340.

［60］黄玲.浅析制霜法的炮制作用［J］.江苏中医药，2004，25（04）：47.

第四章 传统炮制技术工具

中药传统炮制工具包括净制工具、切制工具、炒制工具、蒸煮制工具、其他制法工具和干燥工具等。

一、净制工具

1. 挑选工具

竹匾：将药物放在竹匾内，用于拣去簸不出、筛不下的杂质；或将药材按大小、粗细、长短、厚薄、软硬、颜色等不同档次分类挑选，以便进一步加工。

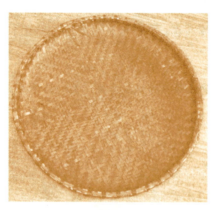

竹匾

2. 筛选工具

根据药物和杂质的体积大小不同，选用不同规格的筛和箩，以筛去药物的砂石、杂质，使其洁净；有些药物形体大小不等，常用不同孔径的筛子进行筛选。

Part II Traditional Processing of Chinese Herbal Medicine

Chapter Four   Traditional Processing Technology Tools

Traditional processing tools of PCHM include cleaning tools, cutting tools, stir-frying tools, cooking tools, other processing tools, and drying tools, etc.

Section One   Cleaning Tools

1. Sorting tools

Bamboo plaque: Crude drugs are placed in the Bamboo plaque to pick out impurities that cannot be dumped or screened. Or the drugs can be sorted and selected according to the different sizes, thickness, length, thickness, hardness, color, and so on, to facilitate further processing.

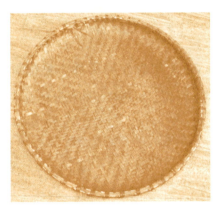

The bamboo plaque

2. Screening tools

According to the volume of drugs and impurities, different sieves and bamboo baskets with different specifications are selected to screen out sands and impurities in drugs to make drugs clean. If drugs vary in size, the sieves with different pore sizes can be applied in screening.

（1）竹筛：圆形浅边，底平有孔，直径50～70cm，四周边高3～4cm，根据筛眼内径大小不同，分为：特大眼筛、大眼筛、中眼筛、谷糠筛、米筛、灰筛。

特大眼筛：习称"附子筛"。规格：筛眼内径28～30mm。常用于摊晾附子、茯苓、大黄等体质粗大的原药材，或作分档用。

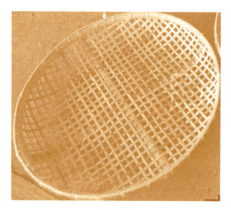

附子筛

大眼筛：习称"禾筛"（相当外地所称"菊花筛"）。规格：筛眼内径16～22mm。常用于川芎、泽泻、川乌等原药材分档或筛去杂质。

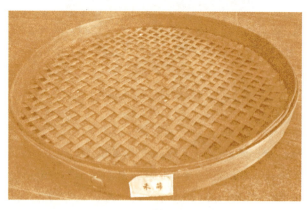

禾筛

(1) The bamboo sieves: Round shallow side, flat bottom with holes, About 50~70 cm in diameter, Peripheral height 3~4cm. Based on the different sizes of the inner meridians of the sieve, the sieves can be divided into extra-large aperture sieves, large-aperture sieves, medium-aperture sieves, grain bran sieves, rice sieves, and ash sieves.

The extra-large-aperture sieve: Commonly known as "Aconiti Lateralis Radix Praeparata (Fuzi) Sieve". The inner diameter sieve opening is 28~30mm. It is often used for spreading and drying the raw big crude drugs with rough texture such as Aconiti Lateralis Radix Praeparata (Fuzi), Poria (Fuling), and Rhei Radix Et Rhizoma (Daihuang), or for grading.

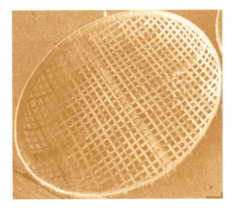

Monkshood Sieve

The large-aperture sieve: Commonly known as "The Grain Sieve" (in a few places, called Chrysanthemum-Juhua sieve). Inner diameter sieve opening is 16 ~ 22mm. It is often used to classify raw drugs according to different sizes or to screen impurities in raw medicinal materials of Chuanxiong Rhizoma (Chuanxiong), Alismatis Rhizoma (Zexie) and Aconiti Kusnezoffii Radix (Chuanwu), etc.

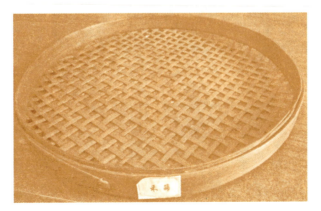

The grain sieve

中眼筛：习称"玄胡筛""半夏筛"。规格：筛眼内径10mm。加工炮制中最为常用，常用于半夏、延胡索、党参、黄芪、山药、炙甘草等药材分档。用固体辅料（糠、麦麸、米等）拌炒片形较大的药材后，多用中眼筛筛去辅料及碎屑。

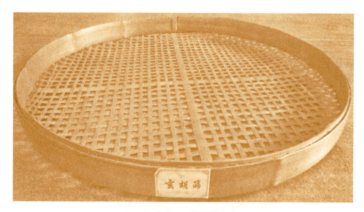

玄胡筛、半夏筛

谷糠筛：糠在用来拌炒药物前，多以其筛去灰屑杂质；用固体辅料拌炒片形较小的药材（如丹参、柴胡、续断、牛膝等）多用谷糠筛筛去辅料及碎屑。规格：筛眼内径5mm。

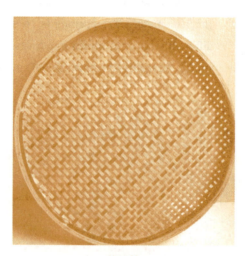

谷糠筛

The medium-aperture sieve: Commonly known as "Corydalis Rhizoma (Yanhusuo) Sieve" and " Corydalis Rhizoma (Banxia) Sieve". The inner diameter sieve opening is 10mm. The most commonly used in processing, such as used in the classification of Pinelliae Rhizoma (Banxia), Corydalis Rhizoma (Yanhusuo), Codonopsis Radix (Dangshen), Astragali Radix (Huangqi), Dioscoreae Rhizoma (Shanyao), Glycyrrhizae Radix Et Rhizoma (Gancao) and other medicinal materials. It is also used to remove the solid assistant materials (grain bran, wheat bran, rice, etc.) or debris in large shape drugs processed by stir-frying with solid assistant materials methods.

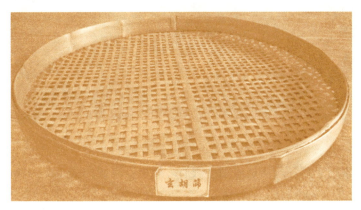

Corydalis Rhizoma (Yanhusuo) sieve & pinelliae Rhizoma (Banxia) sieve

The grain bran sieve: Inner diameter sieve opening is 5mm. Grain bran **sieve** is often used to remove dust impurities mixed in grain bran. It is also used to remove the solid assistant materials (grain bran, wheat bran, rice, etc.) or debris in large shape drugs (such as Salvia Miltiorrhiza Radix Et Rhizoma-Danshen, Bupleuri Radix-Chaihu, Dipsacus Radix-Xuduan, Achyranthis Bidentatae Radix-Niuxi, etc.) processed by stir-frying with solid assistant materials methods.

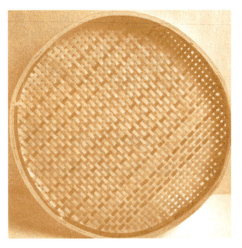

The grain bran sieve

米筛：常用于筛香附米样大小的药材的药屑及中砂、麦麸等固体辅料，亦用于分档和隔去杂质。规格：筛眼内径 3mm。

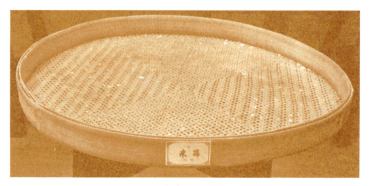

米筛

灰筛：常用于筛各药灰屑或细砂灰屑。规格：筛眼内径 1.5～2mm。

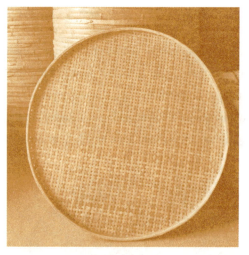

灰筛

以上工具都是用竹篾制成，一般也称"篾筛"。另有一种用于筛去热砂或用于烘焙的筛系极细铁丝制成，习称"铁丝筛"，具有耐高温的特点。

The rice sieve: Inner diameter sieve opening is 3mm. It is commonly used for screening the drug dust in medicinal materials (like Cyperi Rhizoma-Xiangfu) with rice-like size and solid assistant materials, such as sand, wheat bran, etc. And rice sieve is also used to classify drugs of different sizes and remove their impurities.

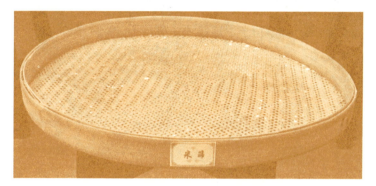

The rice sieve

The ash sieve: Inner diameter sieve opening is 1.5~2mm. It is often used to screen the ash, dust, or fine sand in various drugs.

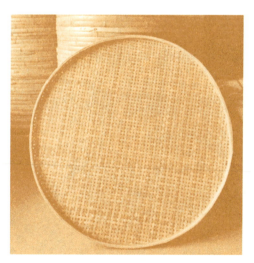

The ash sieve

All the sieves mentioned above are made of bamboo strips, so commonly known as "strip sieve". And another kind of sieve is made of very fine wire, commonly known as "wire sieve", which is used to sieve hot sand or to bake drugs. It has the characteristics of high-temperature resistance.

（2）箩筛：用竹片（或木片）扎成圆筐，筛眼内径比一般筛更小。根据编织筛格材料及罗目大小不同，分为马尾筛、铁丝纱罗、细罗。

马尾筛：也称"马尾筛箩"。由马尾棕织成，故名。现常用尼龙丝织成，称尼龙筛。粗的每 $1cm^2$ 约 3 个眼，细的每 $1cm^2$ 约 5 个眼。主要用于筛颗粒微细的药材中的灰尘、泥灰，如葶苈子、地肤子、菟丝子、蛇床子、天仙子等。

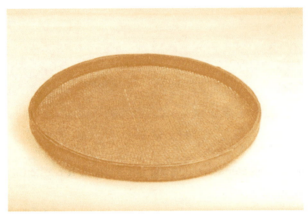

马尾筛

铁丝纱罗：筛底用铁丝纱做成，每 $1cm^2$ 有 1.5～2 个眼。

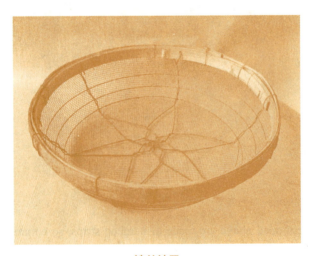

铁丝纱罗

(2) The round sieves: It is a round basket made of the bamboo slice (or wood chip), the inner diameter of the sieve opening is smaller than the general sieve. According to the different weaving materials and sieve opening sizes, the round sieves can be divided into horsetail sieve, wire sieve, and undersize roller.

The horsetail sieve: Also calls "horsetail bamboo sieve". It used to be made of horsetai, and now the weaving material is always nylon yarn, so it is also called "nylon sieve". The relatively large nylon sieve has about 3 sieve opening per 1cm^2 and the relatively fine nylon sieve has about 5 sieve pores per 1cm^2. It is mainly used for sifting the dust or musky coal is relatively small shape drugs, such as Descurainiae Semen Lepidii Semen (Tinglizi), Kochiae Fructus (Difuzi), Cuscutae Semen (Tusizi), Cnidii Fructus (Shechuangzi), and Hyoscyami Semen (Tianxianzi), etc.

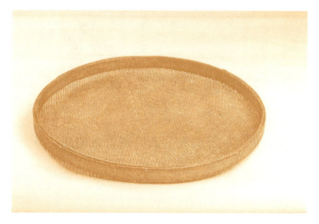

The horsetail sieve

The wire sieve: The bottom of the sieve is made of wire yarn, and there are about 1.5 ~ 2 sieve openings per 1cm^2.

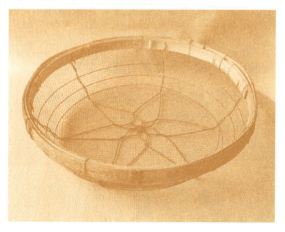

The wire sieve roller

细罗：筛底用丝绢或细铜丝织成，又名"绢筛""铜丝筛"，每 $1cm^2$ 有 8 个眼。主要用于筛取碾槽或乳钵粉碎后的药粉。

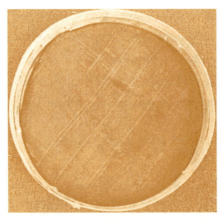

细罗

（3）龟板筛：半球形，底部突起，系以宽竹条编成，每个孔眼相距 1.5～2cm，用于筛体积较大的药物。

（4）套筛：外有圆形木套，上覆以盖，上下两层，中嵌罗筛，全高约 25cm，用套筛的目的主要是使研细的粉末不易飞扬。

有些药物的筛选须用多种罗筛，如花椒的净选：先将花椒倒在灰筛里筛去灰屑，再换中眼筛筛去子（椒目）及残柄细棒，如果有粗梗成串相连的，再用大眼筛过筛，把净椒隔下，把串联在一起的粗梗分开，去棒即可。

3. 风选工具

利用药物和杂质的比重不同，借助风力清除杂质。一般利用簸箕或风车、风扇等通过扬簸或风吹等操作，把不同比重的药材和杂质分开，以达到纯净之目的。如风选莱菔子、葶苈子。

The undersize sieve: The bottom of the sieve is made of tiffany or fine copper wire, also known as "silk sieve", "copper wire sieve", there are about 8 sieve openings per 1cm^2. It is mainly used for screening medicinal powder made by mill groove or mortar.

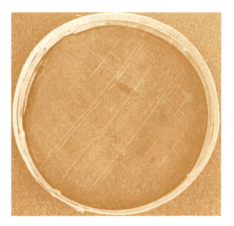

The undersize sieve roller

(3) The tortoise-plastron sieve: The Tortoise-plastron Sieve is hemispherical with a protruding bottom and made of bamboo strips, there is a 1.5 ~ 2cm distance between each sieve opening, and it is used to screen larger shape drugs.

(4) The sieve with outer coat: There is a circular outer coat made with wooden outside the sieve, covered with a lid, showing two layers, the sieve is embodied in the middle, The total height is about 25cm. The purpose to use this tool is to avoid the fine powder flying outside easily.

Some drugs need to be screened with a variety of sieves, such as the selection of Sichuan pepper (Huajiao): firstly, the ash in Sichuan pepper (Huajiao) could be removed with ash sieve, and then the seeds (pepper order) and residual could be removed with medium aperture sieve. If there are thick stems connected in strings remained in drugs, then use a large aperture sieve to separate pure pepper from the thick stems connected in series.

3. Selection with wind

Different proportions of drugs and impurities can be used to remove impurities with the help of wind. Generally, a dustpan or windmill, fan, etc can be used. Through some operations like winnowing or blowing, the medicinal materials and impurities with different specific gravity can be separated to get clean medicinal materials. For example, selecting Cuscutae Semen (Laifuzi), Descurainiae Semen Lepidii Semen (Tinglizi) with the wind.

（1）簸箕：用柳条或竹片制成，利用药物与杂质的不同比重和比例，借上下左右振动簸箕的力量，将杂质簸除、扬净（簸箕和竹匾可以互用）。

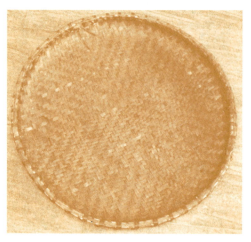

簸箕

（2）风车：木制传统工具，顶部有个梯形的入料仓，下面有一个漏斗是出大米的，侧面有一个小漏斗是出细米、瘪粒的，尾部是出谷壳的；木制的圆形"大肚子"藏有一叶轮，有铁做的摇柄，手摇转动风叶以风扬谷物，转动速度快，产生的风也大。

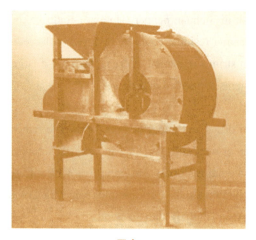

风车

(1) The dustpan: The dustpan is made of wicker or bamboo piece, by the force of upper and lower vibrations of the dustpan, for the different specific gravity of drugs and impurity, the impurity could be removed. (dustpan and bamboo plaque can be used together)

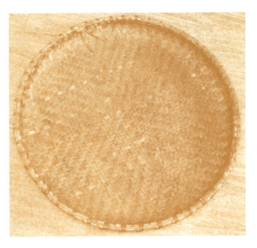

The dustpan

(2) The windmill: The windmill is a traditional wooden tool, with a trapezoidal feeding bin at the top, a funnel at the bottom for discharging rice, a small funnel on the side of the windmill for fine rice and shriveled grain discharging, and the tail part is for the husk discharging. There is an impeller with the iron handle inside the round wooden "big belly" in the middle of the windmill, when turning the impeller with handle, which would produce wind to upwards the grain, and the faster it turns, the greater the wind power is.

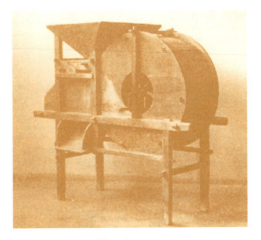

The winnower

（3）扇子：俗称蒲扇。由蒲葵的叶、柄制成，质轻、价廉，是中国应用最为普及的扇子，亦称"葵扇"。除风选药材外，古代在煮药时可用来加大火力。

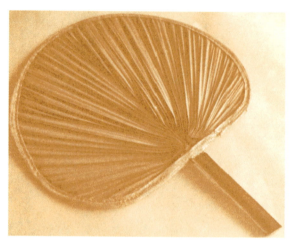

扇子

4. 水选工具

水选是用水冲洗除去杂质，或利用药物与杂质在水中的浮力不同分离非药用部位。

（1）洗净工具：将整理过的药材倒入洗药池内，用清水将药材表面的泥土、灰尘、霉斑或其他不洁之物洗去。洗药池由青砖或椭圆形石头砌成方形或圆形的水池，天然形成的或在石头中间凿出来的水池，用于清洗药材，大小根据药量而定。

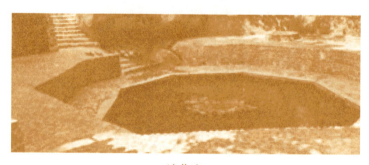

洗药池

(3) The Chinese fan: It is also known as the cattail leaf fan. It is made of the leaves and stalks of the palm anemone, light in weight and cheap, and it is the most popular fan in China, also known as the "palm-leaf fan". In addition, to select drugs with wind, it is also used to increase the fire-power when decocting herbal medicine in ancient times.

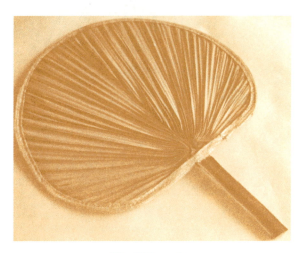

The Chinese fan

4. Selection with water

It is used to remove impurities by washing drugs with water or to separate non-medicinal parts according to the difference of buoyancy between the drugs and the impurities in the water.

(1) Abstersion: It means that putting the selected herbs into the pool for cleaning to wash the dirt, dust, mildew, or other unclean things on the surface of drugs with water. The pool for cleaning is a square or round pool being made of blue brick or oval stone, it can be formed naturally or dig between the stone. It is used for cleaning drugs, the size of the pool depends on the number of the drugs.

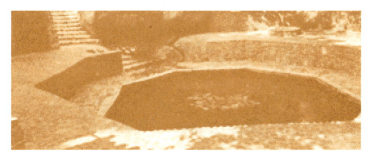

The pool for cleaning

（2）淘洗工具：把药材置于盛器内，用大量清水荡洗附在药材表面的泥沙或杂质。如蝉蜕、蛇蜕。盛器是指盛放东西的器具，竹制或由其他材料制作。

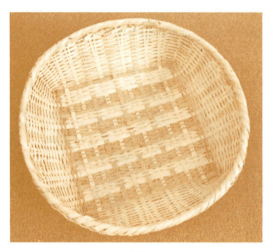

盛器

（3）浸漂工具：将药物置于大量清水中浸较长时间，适当翻动，每次换水；或将药物用竹筐盛好，置于清洁的长流水中漂较长时间，至药材毒质、盐分或腥臭异味得以减除为度，取出干燥，或进一步加工，如乌梅、昆布。常用工具如竹筐。竹筐是竹制工具，用于洗药、润药和装药用。

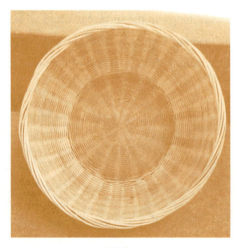

竹筐

(2) Elutriation: It means that putting the drugs in a container, using lots of water to remove the sediment or impurities on the surface of the drugs. Such as the cleaning of Cicada periostracum (Chantui) and Serpentis periostracum (Shetui). The container is an instrument for holding drugs, always made of bamboo or other materials.

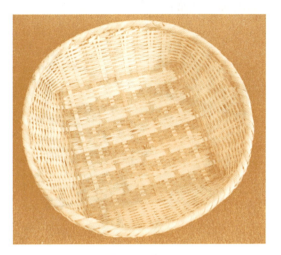

The container

(3) Washing & rinsing: It means to place the drugs in a large amount of clear water and soak it for a long time, with suitable turning and moving, changing the water frequently. Or put the drugs in a bamboo basket in running water for a long time until the toxic components, the salt, or the odor was reduced or removed. Taking out the drugs and making drugs dry or prepare for further processing. For example, the wash and rinse of Mume Fructus (Wumei) and Laminariae Thallus/Ecklonniae Thallus (Kunbu). For the methods, the most used tool is the bamboo basket, which is made of bamboo and used for washing rinsing, and placing drugs.

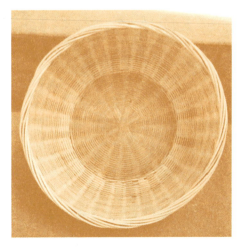

The bamboo basket

5. 其他工具

根据药材质地与性质,传统净制方法还有摘、揉、擦、碃、刷、拭、剪切、挖、刮、剥等。常用工具如碃和刷等。

(1) 碃:用来磨去药物杂质或非药用部分的工具。

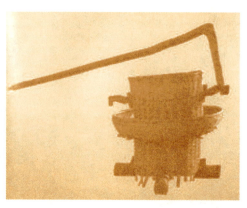

碃

(2) 刷:包括毛刷、尼龙刷或棕榈刷,用于刷去药物外表面灰尘、泥沙、绒毛或其他附着物,如枇杷叶。

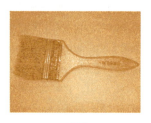  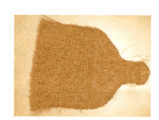

毛刷　　　　　　尼龙刷　　　　　　棕榈刷

5. Other Tools

According to the texture and properties of drugs, the traditional clean methods also include picking, kneading, wiping, husking, brushing, cutting, digging, scraping and peeling, etc. The commonly used tools include.

(1) Husking: It is a tool to grind away the impurities or non-medicinal parts or drugs.

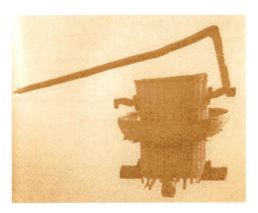

The Husking

(2) Brushing: Including hairbrush, nylon brush, or palm brush, it can be used to brush away dust, dirt, fluff, or other attachments on the surface of drugs, such as brushing the fine hair on the surface of Loquat leaf (Pipaye).

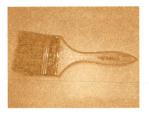  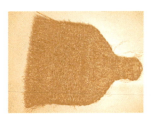

Hairbrush   **Nylon brush**   **Palm brush**

二、切制工具

1. 软化工具

（1）淋法：是将药材整齐堆放，洒壶装清水，从上而下反复浇淋的方法。常用工具有洒壶，为铝制的洒水工具。用于气味芳香、质地疏松的全草、叶、果皮类和有效成分易随水流失的药材的软化。

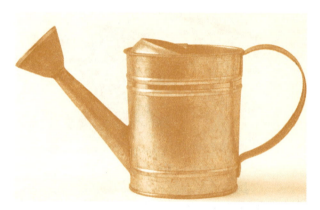

洒壶

（2）淘洗法：用清水洗涤或快速洗涤药材的方法，又称"抢水洗"。常用工具有洗药缸和淘篓。

洗药缸：敞口的大缸，系陶制品，古时用于装水洗药。

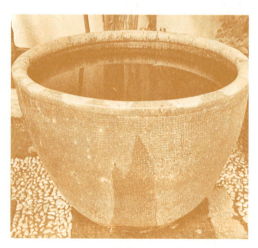

洗药缸

Section Two   Cutting Tools

1. Softening tools

(1) Showering: It means to make herbs being stacked neatly, using a watering pot to pour the herbs from top to bottom repeatedly. The most used tool of the method is the watering pot, which is an aluminum-made sprinkler. It can be used to soften the kinds of grass, leaves, or peel of herbs or those medical materials whose active components are easy to be lost in the water.

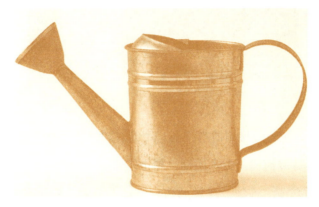

Watering pot

(2) The elutriation method: It means to wash drugs quickly, also known as "washing in a short time". The commonly used tools include washing vat and the basket.

Washing vat: It's pottery, vat without cover. In ancient times it was used to contain water to wash crude drugs.

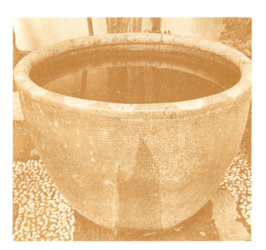

Washing vat

淘篓：为细蔑丝条编织成的能排水的圆箩筐，大量淘洗药材多用淘篓。

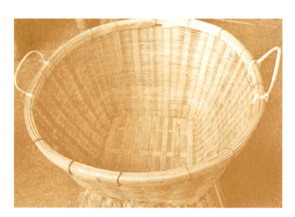

淘篓

（3）浸泡法：是将药材用清水浸泡一定的时间，使其吸收适量水分而软化的方法。常用工具有浸药桶，为木质桶，桶下端近底处设有一放水口，配有木栓。洗、浸、漂油质药或多泡沫、浮屑的药材宜从上放水，粉质或毒性药材从窟洞放水。

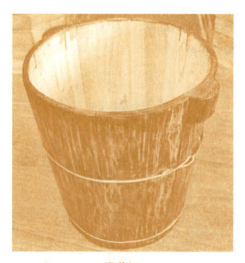

浸药桶

The basket: It was a round basket made of bamboo thin strips. It is capable of draining water and is widely used for the elutriation method.

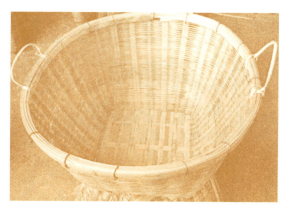

The basket

(3) The immersion method: It means to soak crude drugs with water for a certain period so that the drugs can absorb a suitable amount of water to get soften. The commonly used tool is the immersion bucket which is made of wood. There is a hole in the bottom of the bucket to let the water in or out. The hole was fitted with a wooden cork. If it was used for washing, immersion, or floating drugs containing oil, easily producing foam, or having floating debris, it is proper to add water from the upper of the bucket. If it was used for powdery or toxic herbs, it is better to add water from the bottom hole.

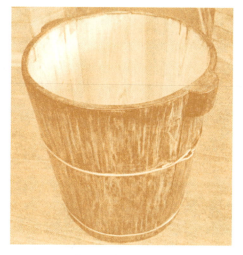

Immersion bucket

（4）**漂法**：是将药材用多量水、多次漂洗的方法。常用工具有笊篱和筲箕。

笊篱：为竹篾编成的打捞工具。适用于洗、泡、浸、漂时打捞药材。

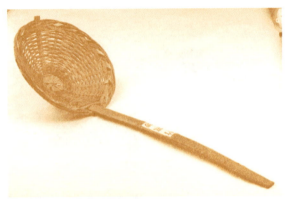

笊篱

筲箕：为竹篾编成的器具。可滤去水液而不流失药材。

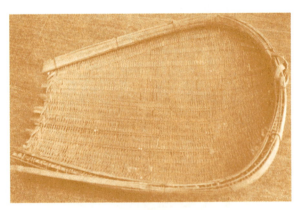

筲箕

(4) The bleaching method: It means to rinse herbs with large amounts of water repeatedly many times. The commonly used tools are bamboo ladle and bamboo strainer.

Bamboo ladle: It is a tool made of bamboo for ladling. It is suitable for ladling herbal medicines in the washing, soaking, or bleaching method.

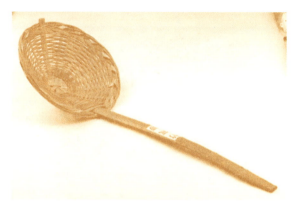

Bamboo ladle

The bamboo strainer: It is an instrument made of bamboo sticks. The water can be filtered through it without the loss of herbal medicines.

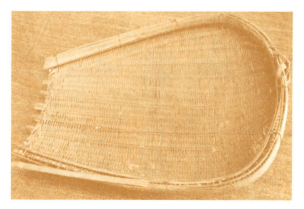

The strainer

（5）润药：是药材水软化最主要的方法，包括浸润、闷润、露润（吸潮回润）。常用工具有润药缸、润药盆、润药丝篓、篾席。

润药缸：为阔口有釉陶器，大小视加工量而定。适宜果实种子、块根药材润制、腌制或饮片闷润（吸收液体辅料）。

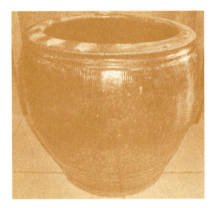

润药缸

润药盆：为小木盆，方便少量润制及复润待切制的药材。必要时上面应用麻布遮盖或加盖。

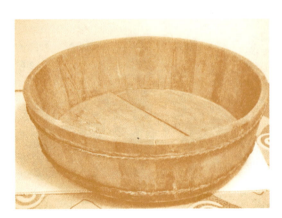

润药盆

(5) The moistening method: It is the most important method of softening herbal medicines with water, the methods including infiltration, smoldering moistening, dew moistening (moisture after absorption of water again). The commonly used tools are moistening cylinder, moistening basin, moistening basket and bamboo mat.

Moistening vat: It is a kind of glazed pottery with a wide mouth, and its size depends on the amount of herbal medicine processed. This vat is suitable for moistening, pickling, and smoldering moistening (for absorption of liquid assistant materials).

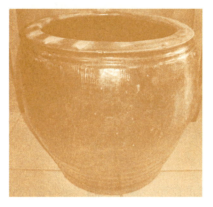

Moistening vat

Moistening basin: It is a small wooden basin and convenient for a small amount of herbal medicine moistening or repeated moistening. If necessary, the linen or lid can be covered on the top of the basin.

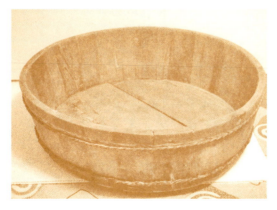

Moistening basin

润药丝篓：为藤、竹或细柳条编织而成，有长方形、圆柱形。大小视加工量而定，适宜抢水洗净药材后，沥干余水，润制药材。

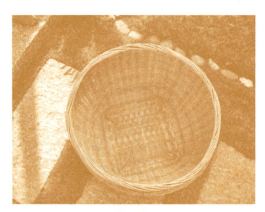

润药丝篓

篾席：为篾片编织成的席子，将含油脂、糖分多的药材，如当归、干地黄等放于垫有篾席或竹垫的湿润土地上，使其自然吸潮回润。

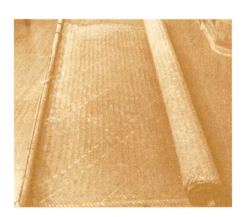

篾席

Moistening wire basket: It is a rectangular or cylindrical basket made of rattan, bamboo, or wicker. Its size depends on the number of herbal medicines processed. It's, suitable for draining the remaining water after cleaning the drugs with lots of water and for moistening either.

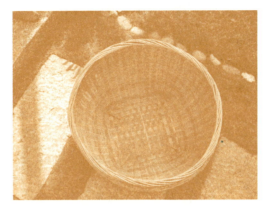

Moistening wire basket

The bamboo mat: It is a mat made of thin bamboo strips. It's suitable for herbal medicines containing many oil and sugar, like Angelicae Sinensis Radix (Danggui) and dried Rehmanniae Radix (Gandihuang). The herbal medicines can be put on the bamboo mat on the wet ground, to get absorption of moisture.

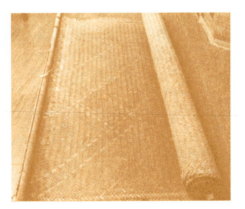

The bamboo mat

2. 切制工具

（1）手工切制：是一种传统加工炮制方法和技巧，是保持中药形、色、气、味的主要技术。所用工具有以下几种。

①铡刀（樟刀）：主要由刀片、刀床（刀桥）、竹压板、木垫、油（水）帚、控药棍等部件组成。多用于铡横薄片，如白芍飞上天、木通不见边等。

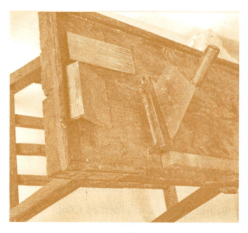

铡刀（樟刀）

②片刀（樟帮）：即类似菜刀、配砧板。樟树铁器厂历来有专用于切药的刀片供应，多用于切厚片、直片、斜片等，如黄芪柳叶片、浙贝元宝片、白术云头片等。

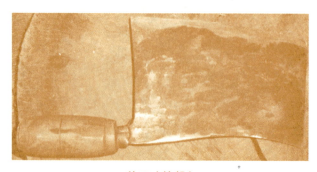

片刀（樟帮）

2. Cutting tools

(1) Manual cutting: As a traditional processing method and technique, it is the main skill to keep the shape, color, and smell of traditional Chinese herbal medicine.

① **The hand hay cutter (Zhangdao):** It is mainly composed of a blade, knife bed (the bridge of knife), bamboo pressure plate, wooden pad, oil (water) broom, control stick, and other parts. This kind of knife is mostly used for cutting horizontal and thin herbal medicine slices, such asPaeoniae Radix Alba (Baishao) which is so thin that can easily be puff to fly to the sky, Akebiae Caulis (Mutong) slices which shows no edge, etc.

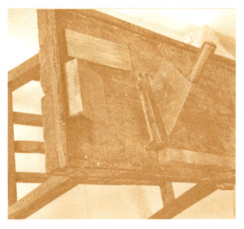

The hand hay cutter (Zhangdao)

② **The sliced knife (belongs to Zhang Society):** It is likely to a kitchen knife Supporting chopping boards Zhangshu city's iron factory has always provided a special blade for cutting herbal medicines slices. This kind of knife is often used to cut herbs into thick slices, straight slices, oblique slices, and so on. Such as willow leaf pieces of the Astragali Radix (Huangqi), Yuanbao like a piece of the Thunberg fritillary bulb (Zhebei), a heap of clouds piece of the Atractylodis Macrocephalae Rhizoma (Baizhu), etc.

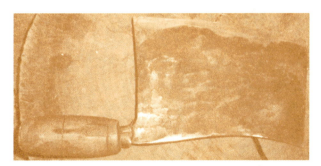

The sliced knife

③铡刀（建昌帮）：药界习称建刀、琢刀、刹刀，其配件有刀案、刀床、苏木刀栓、控药木界尺、油榉、拱形竹夹、竹压板及小条帮刀石等。其中油榉是竹制品，用来给切药刀上油润滑用。刀重约1.5kg，具有刀把长、刀面阔大、刀口线直、刃深锋利、吃硬省力、方便多用等特点。

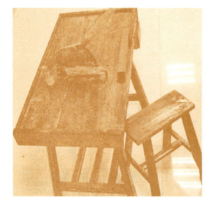

铡刀（建昌帮）

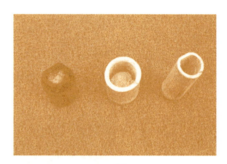

油榉

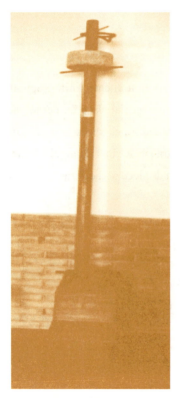

雷公刨（建昌帮）

④雷公刨（建昌帮）：是建昌药界常用的药刨，其加工出的饮片具有"斜、薄、大"的特色。适合刨制长、斜、直、圆各形薄片或极薄片，具片型均匀美观、片张可大可小，工作效率高等特点。过去有专门的刨药师及药工。

③ **The hand hay cutter (belongs to Jianchang Society):** Also known as Jian Chopper, the carving chopper and the chopper like a long spear in traditional. Its fittings include knife case, knife bed, hematoxylon knife bolt, control woody boundary rule, oil beech, arch type bamboo clip, bamboo pressboard, and small strip knife stone, and so on. In the fittings, the oil beech is special, it is made of bamboo and used to lubricate the cutter blade. The knife weighs about 1.5kg and has the characteristics of a long handle, broad blade, straight, deep, and sharp edge, convenient and multi-purpose. It can cut hard things and save energy.

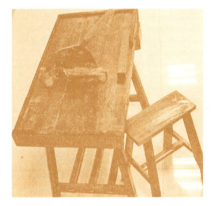

The hand hay cutter (Belongs to Jianchang Society)

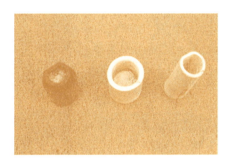

The oiled beech

④ **The leigong sharpener (belongs to Jianchang Society):** It is commonly used in Jianchang Society. And the processed slices have the characteristics of slanting, thin and big. It is suitable for cutting long, oblique, straight, and round slices or extremely thin slices. The characteristic of the tool is the cut pieces are even and beautiful, the area of the piece can big or small, and the working efficiency is high. In the past, there were specialized planers and pharmacists to use this tool.

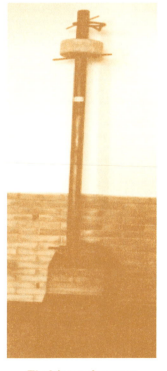

The leigong sharpener (Belongs to Jianchang Society)

⑤**磨刀石**:磨刀的传统工具。石有四种,按石头质地和磨刀工序中运用的先后顺序排列为:红石、猪肝色磨刀石、青磨刀石、小条帮刀石。

红石(红糙石):石质粗糙、摩擦力大,适用于新刀开口、磨去右面余铁、刀口缺损须快速磨去缺痕。

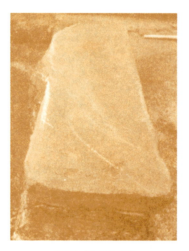

红石(红糙石)

猪肝色磨刀石(猪肝石):以石为猪肝色为名,石质细嫩,石面平坦且坚硬,磨刀粉浆重,涩性大、吃铁多、易薄口、磨刀速度快。是建昌帮主要刀石,多为广昌县所产。

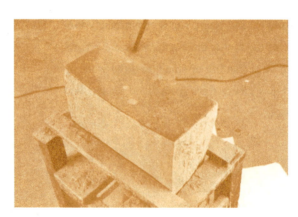

猪肝色磨刀石(猪肝石)

⑤ **The sharpening stone:** The sharpening stone is a traditional tool for sharpening knives. There are four kinds of sharpening stones. According to the texture of stone and the sequence of the knife used during the grinding process, it can be divided into, red stone, pig-liver sharpening stone, blue sharpening stone, small sharpening stone.

The red stone (red rough stone): This stone is rough with high friction. It is suitable for a new knife to put the first edge, grinding the remained iron on the right side of a knife, and quickly grinding the missing mark on the edge of a knife.

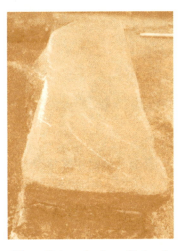

The red stone (red rough stone)

The pig-liver sharpening stone (liver stone): This is named for the color of the stone (Showed liver color). The stone is delicate, flat, hard, and with big mealiness, and easy to sharpen the edge of the knife and grind quickly. It is the main sharpening stone in Jianchang Society, mostly produced in Guangchang city.

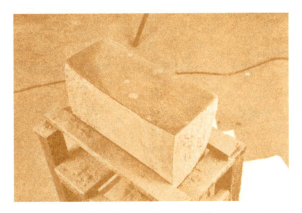

The pig-liver sharpening stone (liver stone)

青磨刀石：石质光亮嫩滑，石面平坦且尤其坚硬，石型同猪肝石，适应用于猪肝石开口后磨出刃口现青光的刀锋，并可使切片光滑平整、无刀痕。

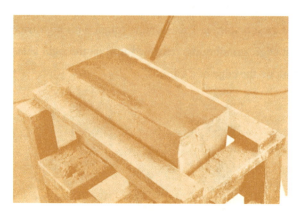

青磨刀石

小条帮刀石：系刀案上切药时，随时用来帮刀起锋的工具。

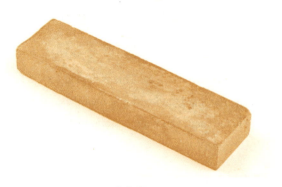

小条帮刀石

磨刀工具配件：大盆（盛盐水置磨刀石架左侧）；蘸水布帚（木把上扎有布条的布帚）。

The blue sharpening stone: The stone is bright and smooth, with a flat and especially hard surface. The stone type is the same as a pig-liver sharpening stone. It is suitable for the cutting edge with blue light after being grinding with pig liver stone and can make the slice smooth and flat without showing a knife mark.

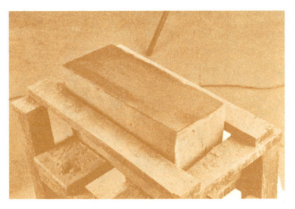

The blue sharpening stone

The small sharpening stone: It is always put on the knife table, it is a tool used to help the blade keeping sharp at any time during cutting.

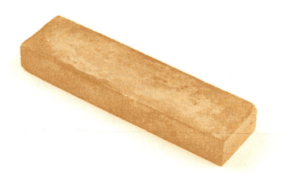

The small side sharpening stone

The accessories for sharpening also include: the big basin (put on the left side of sharpening stone frame with salt water), A cloth brush with water (a broom with clothes on a wooden handle)

⑥特殊加工工具

竹笼撞毛器：又称"香附笼""撞笼"，为竹篾制的撞毛长竹笼。竹笼大小根据药材加工量而定。其形状为梭形，两头尖，中部膨隆。笼体由长条厚黄篾编织而成，笼体中有数根主筋贯穿两头，主筋由略粗竹片及竹竿构成。正中上方开有一方窗，窗上设有活动篾门。两端尖部各设有两个木把手，方便两手握持。

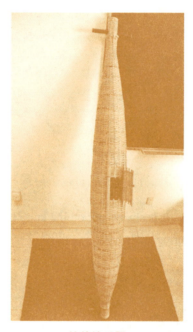

竹笼撞毛器

枳壳夹：是枳壳挖去内瓤后初步定型的工具，为铁制品，安装在长条凳上，下面一块叫夹板床，由角铁改制成，直角在右下方，竖边可拦阻压扁的枳壳肉不向外溢出，使压边均匀，上面一块叫活动夹板，近身端有小木把。

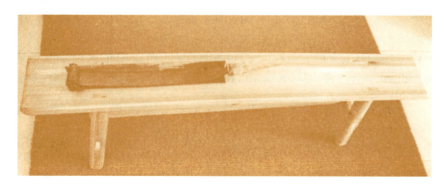

枳壳夹

⑥ The tools for special processing

The bamboo cage used to remove hair: It is a long bamboo cage made of bamboo strips, which is also known as "Cyperi Rhizoma (Xiangfu) cage" or "collision cage". The size of the bamboo cage is determined according to the processing amount of medicinal materials, and its shape is fusiform, two ends are pointed and the middle is swelled. The cage is made of long thick yellow strips. Several main tendons are running through both ends of the cage that composed of slightly thick bamboo slices and bamboo poles. In the middle of the upper part of the bamboo cage, there is a window with a movable gate. And two wooden handles are arranged at the tip of each end for easy holding.

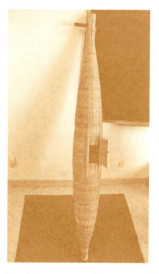

The bamboo cage used to remove hair

The Aurantii Fructus (Zhiqiao) clip: The Fructus aurantii clip is a preliminary shaping tool for Fructus aurantii after removing the inner pulp. It is made of iron and fixed on a long bench, a plywood bed with a right angle is under the clip, which is made of angle iron. The purpose of the bed is to keep the crushed Fructus auranti flesh from spilling out and make the edges even. There is a movable splint on the top of the clip, with a small wooden handle at the close end.

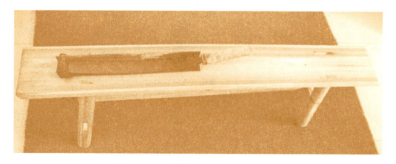

The Aurantii Fructus (Zhike) clip

枳壳榨：是长方形梯式枳壳定型工具。由榨柱、榨板、斧型楔、固定板组成。擎起各层上榨板，将打扁的枳壳整齐平叠在内，叠满为止，然后将上榨板压下，以两边榨柱正面上方通洞中打进斧型楔，榨紧。

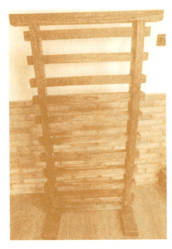

枳壳榨

蟹爪钳：为具有弹性之薄铁条制成，上下对折，前端部有锯齿形咬口，宽约寸余，长约5寸，为切药时钳夹药物之用。用来加工有些"个活"，如槟榔，可用"蟹爪钳"夹紧向前推进。

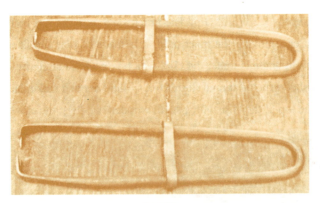

蟹爪钳

Press tool for Aurantii Fructus (Zhike): It is a rectangular ladder shape for initial finalization for Fructus aurantii. It is composed of the press column, the press plank, ax-type wedge, and fixed plate. When operating, lifting the pressing plates on each layer, and arrange many flattened Fructus aurantii neatly between the two plates until they are full. And then pressing down the upper press plate and squeeze with pressing ax-shaped wedges into the upper holes on both sides.

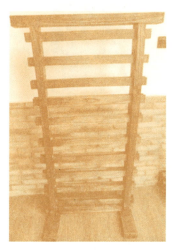

Press tool for Aurantii Fructus (Zhike)

The crab claw pliers: It is a tool made of elastic thin iron bars, folded up and down, in the front part there is a serrated bite, about 3 cm wide. The plier is about 15cm long and suitable for catching drugs when cutting. The crab claw pliers are used to process some "medicinal materials not easy to grasp", such as Areca catechu (Binglang). It can be used to grasp the drugs tightly and make drugs forward to the cutter's edge for best cutting.

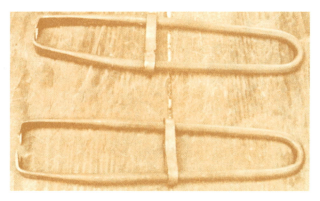

The crab claw pliers

鹿茸加工壶：为加工鹿茸特制的常用工具。

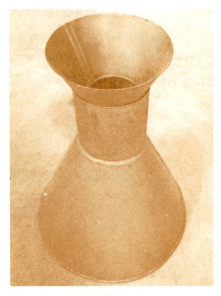

鹿茸加工壶

槟榔榉：为建昌帮切制槟榔的特殊常用工具。木质，长 7cm，上面为圆拱形，下面为平面，右面大头截面中心内凹为圆锅状，凹面内嵌以三颗铁针，针尖平截面以品字形排列，针体棱形，上尖下略粗。

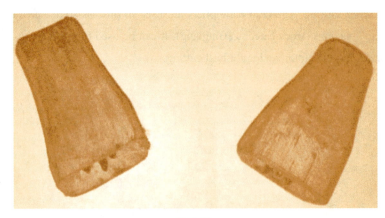

槟榔榉

The Velvet antler (Lurong) processing pot: It is a common tool specially made for processing the Velvet antler.

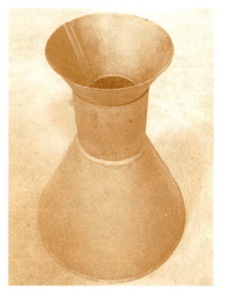

The Velvet antler (Lurong) processing pot

Holder for Areca catechu (Binglang): It is a special and commonly used tool for cutting Areca catechu in Jianchang Society. It is made of wood, 7cm long, showing a round arch above and plan below. The section center of its right is concave into a round shape, in it, there are three iron needles, arranged by an equilateral triangle. The needles show slightly thicker on the top and slightly coarse on the end.

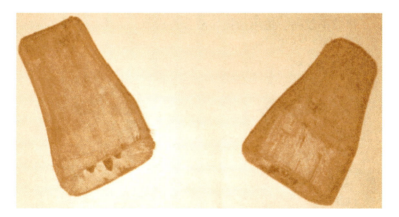

Holder for Areca catechu (Binglang)

三角药架：木制，用于放置竹匾、箩盖、竹筛，以及摊晾药材或饮片。

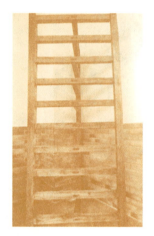

三角药架

（2）其他切制：其他切制法用到的工具有以下几种。

镑刀：为一种特制的镑片工具，为一块厚木板上平行镶嵌多个平行的刀片，两端有控手的木柄，用于角质类药材镑成极薄片，如羚羊角、水牛角等。

刨刀：又称药刨，适合刨制长、斜、直、圆各形薄片或厚片。刨刀结构类似木工刨刀。使用时将刨刀斜固定在木凳上，用平木板或特制药斗压住润好的药材，在刨面上来回推动，即可将药材刨成薄片，刨片片型美观，片张可大可小，可薄可厚，工作效率较高。适用药物如檀香、松节、苏木、牛角等。

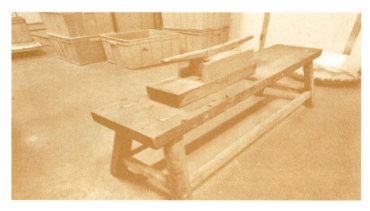

刨刀

The triangle medicine frame: It is made of wood, used for placing bamboo tablets, basket cover, bamboo sieves, drying herbs or pieces.

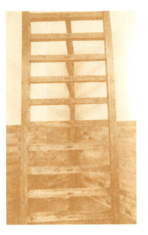

The triangle medicine frame

(2) Other Cutting Tools: There are several tools used in other chelation methods.

The flaker: The Knife is a special cutting tool consisting of parallel blades on a thick plank, with a handle at each end. It is used to cut horny medicines into very thin slices, for example, cutting Saigae Tataricae Cornu (Lingyangjiao) and Buffalo horn (Shuiniujiao) into very thin slices.

The planer: Also known as medicine planer. It is suitable for planing long, oblique, straight, round slices or thick slices. The structure of the planer is similar to that of the wood planer. And when in use, fix the planer knife on the wooden stool obliquely, use the flat board or the special medicine bucket to hold the moistened medicinal materials. The medicinal materials can be planed into thin slices by pushing them back and forth on the planing surface. The slices are beautiful in the shape of large or small, thin or thick. The efficiency of planning is very high. For example, the planting of Sandalwood (Tanxiang), Loose knot (Songjie), Hematoxylin (Sumu), and Ox horn (Niujiao).

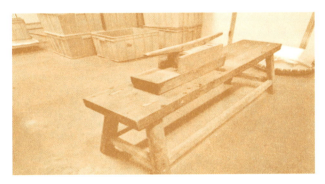

The planer tool

锉刀：锉刀表面上有许多细密刀齿，条形，用于部分习惯上用粉末且用量小、未事先准备、随处方加工的药材，如水牛角、羚羊角等。

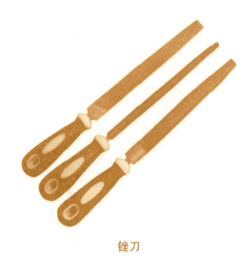

锉刀

劈刀：重约 0.5kg，刀背厚、背与刀口呈三角形者又称"劈斧"，成长条形者又称"镰刀"。主要用于劈切坚硬木质类药材，如檀香、降香、松节等。

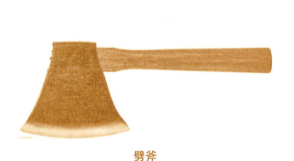

劈斧

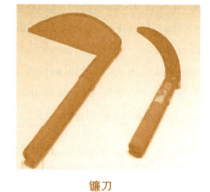

镰刀

The file: There is a lot of fines and dense cutter tooth on the surface of the file. It is used for some Ad-hoc processing herbs which are usually taken in powder with a small dosage, such as Saigae Tataricae Cornu (Lingyangjiao) and Buffalo horn (Shuiniujiao).

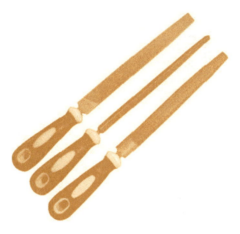

The file

The chopper: It weighs about 0.5kg, the knife back is thick, and the back and edge show a triangle shape, also called "split ax". The one with a long strip is called "sickle". The chopper is mainly used for chopping hard woody herbs, such as Sandalwood (Tanxiang), Rosewood heart-wood (Jiangxiang), and Loose knot (Songjie).

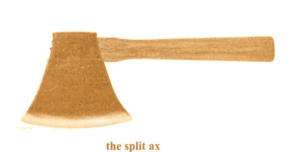

the split ax

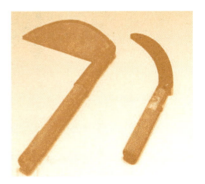

the sickle

剪刀：主要用于剪枝梗、绳索。

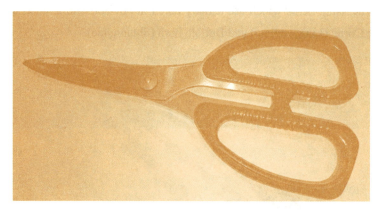

剪刀

茯苓刀：又称靴型皮刀，刀口薄，主要用于铲削茯苓皮等。另有茯苓钻，用以检查润制时药材软化程度。

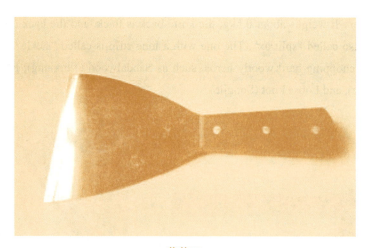

茯苓刀

Part II Traditional Processing of Chinese Herbal Medicine

Scissors: The scissors are mainly used for pruning stem and rope.

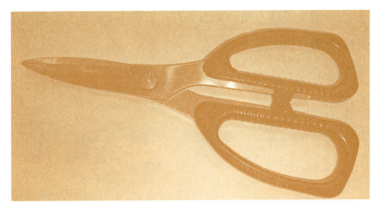

scissors

The Poria (Fuling) shovel: Also known as the boot-type leather knife, its blade is thin. It is mainly used for scooping and peeling Poria peels. Additionally, there is also a Poria drill which is used to check the degree of softening of herbal medicines during moistening.

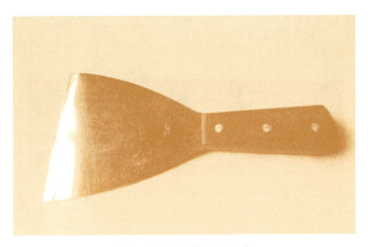

The Poria (Fuling) shovel

竹茹刀：形狭长微弯，具有双柄，上方为刀背，下方为刀口，长约1.2尺，宽约3寸，专为刮取竹茹用。

麦冬刀：为一般小刀或刀面略宽的小刀，主要用于麦冬去心制勺片，以及刮去动物类药材的筋膜残肉。

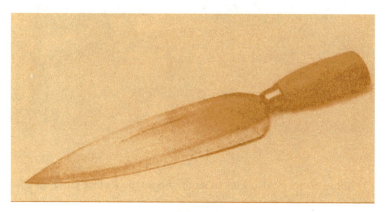

麦冬刀

铜刀、竹刀：铜刀主要用于各种忌铁药材，如熟地黄等。忌铜、铁者用竹刀。

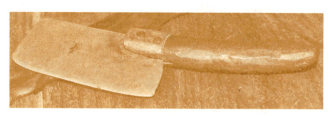

铜刀

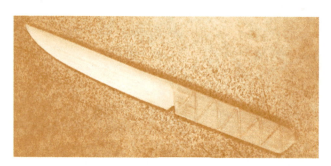

竹刀

Bambusae Caulis in Taenia (Zhuru) knife: It is narrow, long, and slightly curved with double handles. The upper part is the back of the knife and the lower part is the blade. It is about 40cm long and 10cm wide, it is specially used for scraping bamboo shavings.

Radix Ophiopogonis (Maidong) knife: It is a general small knife or a knife with a wider blade. It is mainly used to remove the heart of Radix ophiopogonis and scrape off the fascia residue of animal medicines.

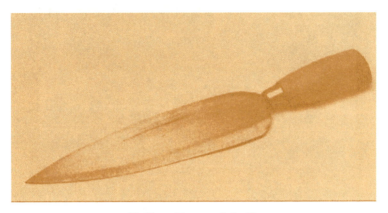

Radix ophiopogonis knife

The copper knife & the bamboo knife: Copper knife is mainly used in all kinds of medicinal materials which are anti-iron, such as prepared Rehmannia root (Shudihuang). Bamboo knives are used in medicinal materials that are anti-iron or anti-copper.

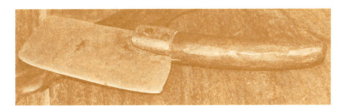

The copper knife

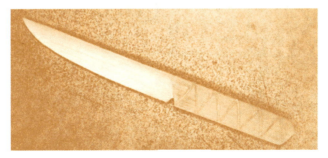

The bamboo knife

刮刀：刮去毛，刮去药物表面的毛绒物，主要用于比较硬的药物，如马钱子等。

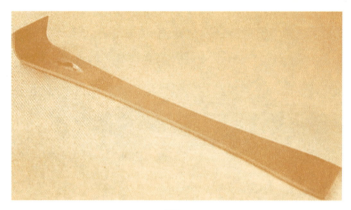

刮刀

碾槽：由生铁铸成，分研槽、研盘两部分。研槽中部阔大，两端狭窄，里面凹形如船，大小不一；研盘为扁圆形铁饼，中心贯有铁杠，突出两旁，操作时两足踏其上前后转动，使药物通过推研而粉碎。

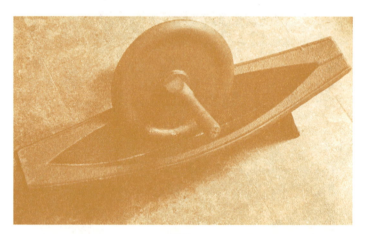

碾槽

The scraper knife: Its function is to scrape off the fluff from the surface of the drugs, mainly for the comparatively hard drugs, such as Strychni Semen (Maqianzi).

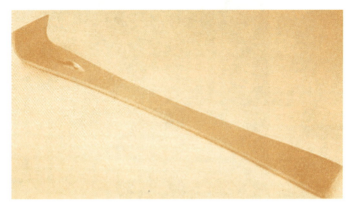

The scraper knife

The mill groove: It is made of cast iron, and consists of two parts: the grinding trough and the pestle. The middle part of the grinding trough is broad, and the two ends are narrow, which are not of uniform size, look like a boat. The pestle is an oblate circle discus, the center of it is perforated with an iron bar to protrude both sides. when operating, the feet step on the bar to make the pestle turn back and forth to make the herbal medicines grind and smash.

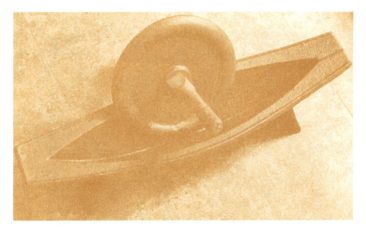

The mill groove (for crushing)

铜冲：又称"冲钵"，身为铜制品，钵有一牛皮盖（铜盖较多见），盖中心有一圆洞，锤穿洞而过插入钵中。

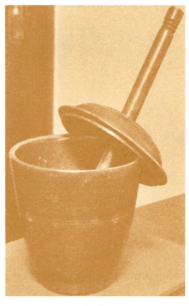

铜冲

石臼：是用粗糙的大石块凿成，方形或圆形，中有凹窝，配有大木槌，粉碎药物。主要用于忌铜、铁药物的捣碎或捣末。

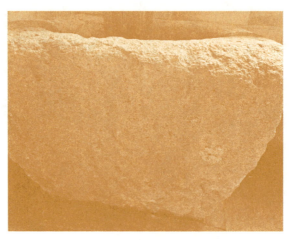

石臼

The copper flush: Also known as "Chong bowl". It is made of copper. There is a cowhide cover (more common is copper cover) on the pot and a round hole in the center of the cover, the hammer goes through the hole and into the bowl to crush herbal medicines.

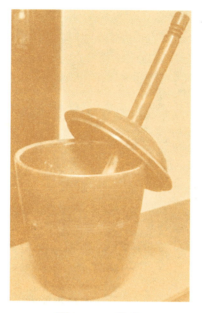

The copper flush

The stone mortar: It is a square or round mortar being made of rough large stones. There is a slot in the middle of the mortar. A big wooden hammer is used when crushing the drugs. It is mainly used for pounding drugs to pieces or crushing drugs which are anti-copper or anti-iron.

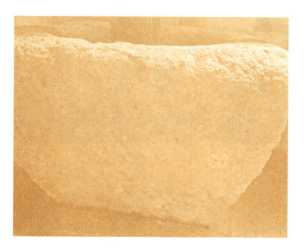

The stone mortar

石磨：是把药物去皮或研磨成粉末的石制工具。由两块尺寸相同的短圆柱形石块和磨盘构成。

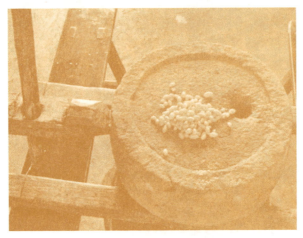

石磨

石碾：系石制成的圆形大磨盘，上置圆柱形滚筒，磨盘与滚筒表面均凿有横棱纹，盘的一方略低，开一小孔，当药物被粉碎后，便从小孔处漏下。

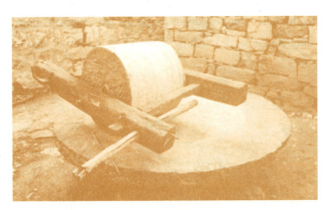

石碾

Part II Traditional Processing of Chinese Herbal Medicine

The stone mill: It is a stone tool used for peeling or grinding herbal medicines. It consists of two short cylindrical blocks of the same size and a grinding wheel.

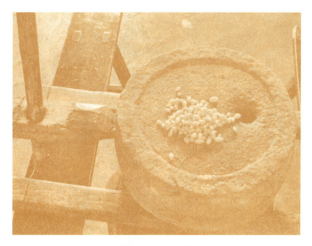

The stone mill

The kollergang: It is a large round grinding disc made of stone, with a cylindrical roller on top. The surface of the grinding disc and the roller are both chipped with transverse ridges, and one side of the disc is slightly lower with a small hole. After the drugs are crushed, they will be leaking through the hole.

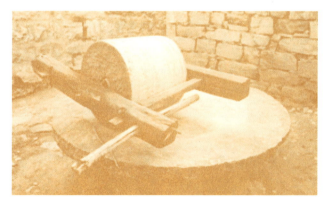

The kollergang

擂钵：适用于少量细料药物研极细药末。

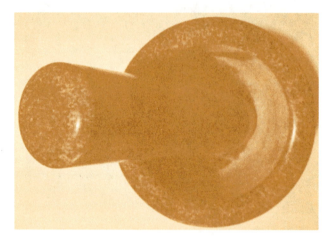

擂钵

铁锤：适用于某些药材敲碎或打成小片，如龟板、鳖甲。

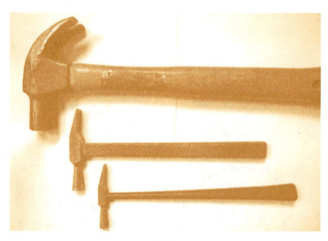

铁锤

The grinding bowl: It is suitable for grinding a small amount of fine material medicine to a very fine powder.

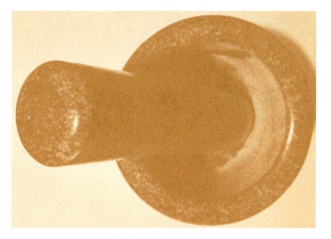

The grinding bowl

The hammer: It is suitable for crushing some medicinal materials or beating them into small pieces. Such as Testudinis Plastrum (Guiban), Trionycis Carapax (Biejia).

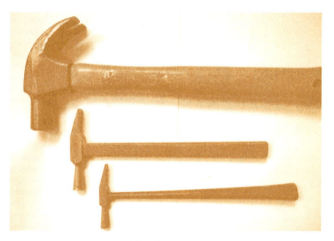

The hammer

铲刀（香附铲）：为木把铁制双片或三片铲刀，主要用于铲切香附米等。

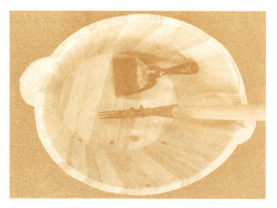

铲刀（香附铲）

三、炒制工具

1. 锅及配件

（1）锅：作为炒制工具的锅有铁锅、铜锅、不锈钢锅之分。

铁锅：铁锅有生铁锅和熟铁锅两种，蒸、煮、熬用的一般为生铁锅，炒、炙用的宜熟铁锅。生铁锅有锅大底深，容药量大的特点，但传热稍慢且易破裂。熟铁锅有锅小底浅，传热快，不易破裂的特点。

鉴别铁锅质量，主要看铁色的光泽。生铁锅以色青发亮为优；熟铁锅以白亮为优，暗黑较差。此外，还要看有无砂眼及裂缝等。

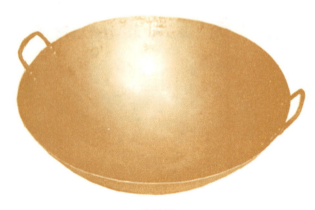

生铁锅

The shovel (Cyperi Rhizoma-Xiangfu shovel): It is a shovel with two or three pieces of iron blades and a wooden handle. It is mainly used for shoveling Cyperi Rhizoma.

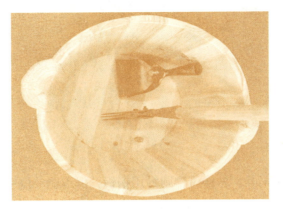

Cyperi Rhizoma shovel

Section Three   Frying Tools

1. Pot & accessories

(1) The pot: The pot can be divided into an iron pot, copper pot, and stainless steel pot.

The iron pot: There are two kinds of iron pot, a cast iron pot, and a wrought iron pot. The cast iron pot is always used for the steaming or boiling process, the wrought iron pot is commonly used for stir-frying or stir-frying with liquid assistant materials process. The cast iron pot is with deep bottom and has a large capacity, slower heat transferring, and easier to break compared to the wrought iron pot, which is small with a shallow bottom, fast heat transfer, and not easy to break.

To identify the quality of the iron pot, the luster of the pot is very important. The cast iron pot has a bright green color, the wrought iron pot has white bright for the best, dark for the worst. In addition, there should not have a sand hole and crack.

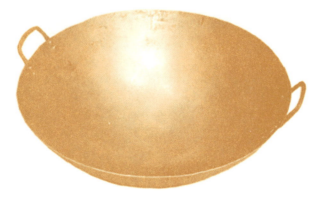

The cast iron pot

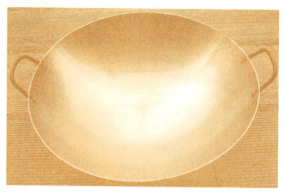

熟铁锅

铜锅：即铜制锅具。忌铁药物则另用铜锅，但不能一概用铜锅。李时珍有"铜器盛饮食茶酒，经夜有毒，煎汤饮，损人声音"之说，并为科学所证实。

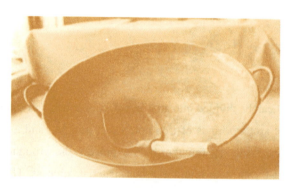

铜锅

不锈钢锅：为不锈钢制工具，现代常用于各种药物的炮制。

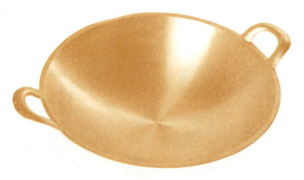

不锈钢锅

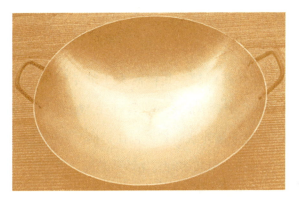

The wrought iron pot

The copper pot: It means the tool is made of copper. The copper pot is used for some herbal medicines that are anti-iron, not all of them. Li shizhen used to say that "the tea or wine put in copperware through one night will be poisonous and if the tea or wine was further cooked with the copperware, it will damage people's vocal cords after drinking", which has been confirmed by scientific study.

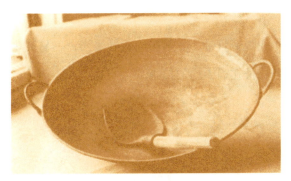

The copper pot

The stainless steel pot: It is stainless steel tool. It is used for many processing methods nowadays.

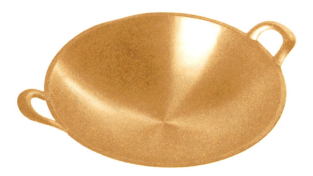

The stainless steel pot

（2）配件

炒药铲：药界又称炒药锅铲。其铲面大于炒菜锅铲，铲面宽 13cm，长 17cm，铲面两侧略卷起，铲柄管长 5cm，管外径 17cm，柄与铲面有时成 150° 角。老药工习惯用粗纸卷成漏斗状防护罩包住铲柄，方便急火快炒时手不被烫伤。药材质重、体大、片厚；量较多时宜用炒药铲翻炒。

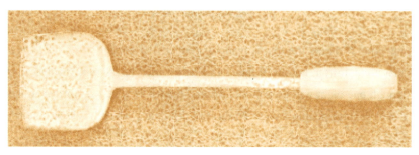

炒药铲

炒药扫帚：为小兜观音笤帚，其茎粗细软硬妥当，不易被热锅烫坏。药材质轻、量少时可用炒药扫帚在锅中均匀扫刷。

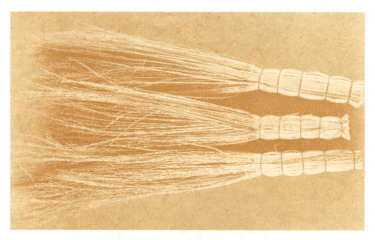

炒药扫帚

(2) Accessories

The frying shovel of herbal medicines: It is also called the frying spatula of herbal medicines. The shovel surface is 13cm wide and 17cm long. Both sides of the shovel are slightly rolled up. The handle pipe is 5cm long. The outside diameter of the pipe is 17cm, the handle and the spatula surface form an angle of 150°. The experienced medicine workers are used to put the rolled thick paper on the below half of the handle to avoid being burned during stir-frying. It is suitable for stir-frying some heavy, big, and thick herbal medicines slices in large numbers.

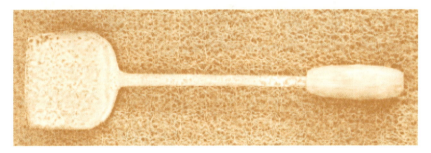

The frying shovel of herbal medicines

The frying broom of herbal medicines: It's a little pocket broom made of Bambusa multiplex with the right stem. It is not easy to be damaged by a hot pot. It's suitable for stir-frying some light herbal medicine slices in small quantities. When stir-frying, using the broom to brush the slices equably in the pot.

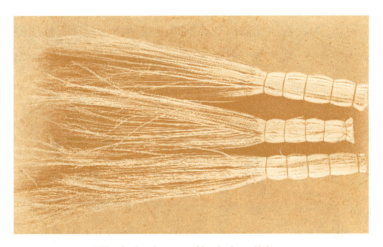

The frying broom of herbal medicines

撮斗：有蔑质与铁质两种，另有手提撮斗。铁撮斗具耐高温的特点，适用于砂炒药物出锅。

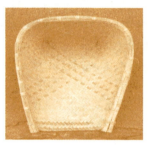 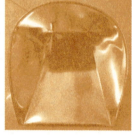 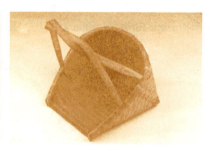

撮斗　　　　　铁撮斗　　　　　手提撮斗

2. 灶

灶是炮制时加热的设施。药师必须熟悉灶的基本知识，才能正确地运用各种火候，炮制出形、色、气、味俱佳的饮片。一般有斜面灶、塘锅灶、炉灶、围灶、老虎灶五种。

（1）斜面灶：为状若鸡囚（鸡窝、鸡舍）的立式灶，故又称"鸡囚灶"。多用于炒、炙等火制法用的铁锅，锅口 52～60cm，锅口一边离近身侧灶边缘 6cm，锅底不宜太深。铁锅斜嵌在灶上，故称"斜锅灶"。

（2）塘锅灶：为状若池塘的锅灶。锅口平或稍高于地面，锅底深凹低于地面，故又称"平面灶"。蒸、煮、熬等水火共制用的，锅宜平嵌灶上，锅口宜大，直径约 67cm 以上。锅底宜深，含水量才多。

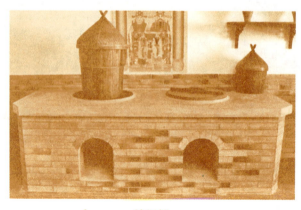

塘锅灶

The winnowing fan: There are two kinds of the tool, being made of viscid or iron. There's still another kind of winnowing fan with a handle. The iron winnowing fan has high-temperature resistance and is suitable for the processing method of stir-frying slices with sand.

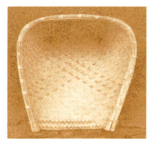 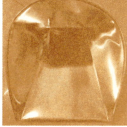 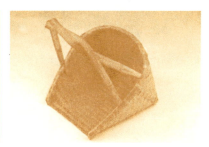

The winnowing fan　　　　The iron winnowing fan　　　　The winnowing fan with handle

2. The Cooking range

The cooking range is a facility for heating during processing. Pharmacists must be familiar with the basic knowledge of the cooking range, to correctly control the fire heating to process the right herbal medicine slices with good shape, color, and smell. There are five different types of cooking range, including oblique cooking range, pond cooking range, stoves, enclosed cooking range, and tiger cooking range.

(1) The oblique cooking range: It is an upright cooker with the shape of a chicken coop, so it is also known as a "chicken stove". The iron pots with stir-frying processing method are used in this range. The mouth of the pot is 52~60 cm, one side of the pot mouth is 6 cm away from the edge of the range side. The bottom of the pot should not be too deep. For the iron pot is obliquely embedded in the range, it is also called "oblique cooker range".

(2) The pond cooking range: It is a cooking range with the shape of a pond. The mouth of the pot is flat or slightly above the ground, and the bottom of the pot is lower than the ground, so it is also called "plane cooking range". The pot needs to be horizontally embedded on the stove when processing herbal medicines with steaming, boiling, and decocting The pot mouth should be large with a diameter of more than 67 cm. The bottom of the pot should be deep enough to contain more water.

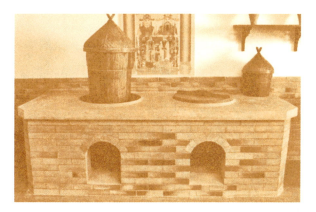

The pond cooking range

（3）炉灶：为大小各种型号风炉，又称"泥炉"。适合药店临时小炒和少量煅药用。用时只要将铁锅架于炉灶上。另有一种炼丹炉灶，为冶炼各种丹药用。

（4）围灶：为临时以砖砌成四围或三围（一方靠墙）的灶圈。圈围内空及高度视制药量而定。建造地点以避风雨处、坐北朝南为宜。适用于煨制、炆制、煅制药物，具有火力集中，避风防火灾的作用。

（5）老虎灶：形似卧虎的长型连锅灶，灶门如虎头，向上仰起。进燃料口如虎口，向上张口。靠地凹下部分是通风口和燃料烧尽后的出灰口，灶尾为烟囱，有数米高。此灶的主要燃料为粗糠和木屑，该灶适用蒸、煮、熬等多种药材的炮制，而且火力大，易控制温度。

3. 火候

（1）不同火源：《本草纲目》将火分成燧火、桑柴火、炭火、阳火与阴火、芦火与竹火、艾火、神针火、火针、灯火、灯花、烛烬等，各种火源功用亦有差异。如栎炭火宜锻炼一切金石药物；陈芦、枯竹之火，取其不强，不损药力；桑柴火能助药力。

竹火：传统炮制热源之一。竹子燃烧之火。取其火力不强，不损药力。

芦火：传统炮制热源之一。指芦苇燃烧之火。取其火力不强，不损药力。

柳木火：系指用柳枝作燃料的炮制热源。既有柳木火，也有柳木炭火、柳木炭等。

炭火：即木炭燃烧之火。栎炭火宜锻炼一切金石药。

桑柴火：传统炮制热源之一。桑树燃烧之火。制备补药、煎熬诸膏多用桑柴火。

糠灰火：又称糠灰、糠火、灰火，为柴草燃烧时未熄灭的细灰烬。适用于"炮"或"煨"制药物。

(3) **The tove:** It consists of all sizes of the stove, also known as "mud stove". It is suitable for temporary stir-frying herbal medicines with low heat and calcining herbal medicines in a small amount. Place the iron pot on the stove when needed. There is another kind of alchemy stove just for smelting various Dan medicines

(4) **The enclosed stove:** It is a kind of brick stove that is four or three sides (one side against the wall) enclosed when needed. The volume of enclosed range and height of the stove is decided by the amount of drug. The stove should be sheltered from wind and rain and oriented south. It is suitable for the processing methods of roasting, braising, and calcining. The function of this stove is to concentrate firepower, avoid wind and prevent fire.

(5) **The tiger stove:** It's a long stove with a pot and the shape of the stove is like a lying tiger. The stove door is like the tiger head that raises. The fuel inlet is like a tiger's mouth opening up. The concave part is the air vent and ash outlet, the end of the stove is a chimney several meters high. The main fuel of the stove is coarse bran and sawdust. It is suitable for the processing methods of steaming, boiling, and decocting. The characteristic of the stove is high heating and temperature control

3. The duration and degree of heating

(1) **Different sources of fire:** In *The Compendium of Materia Medica* (*Bencao Gangmu*), the fire is divided into flint fire, mulberry fire, charcoal fire, Yang fire and Yin fire, reed fire and bamboo fire, mugwort fire, god needle fire, fire needle, candle flame, snuff, and candle ember, etc. The functions of various fires are different. For example, an oak charcoal fire is suitable for calcining all kinds of metals and minerals in medicine. Dried reed and dried bamboo fires are not so strong that they would not damage the effects of medicines. Mulberry fire can assist the effect of medicines.

The bamboo fire: One of the traditional processing heat sources. It's the fire that burning bamboo, which is not so strong as to damage the effect of medicines.

The reed fire: One of the traditional processing heat sources. It's the fire that burning reed, which has the same effect as the bamboo fire.

The willow fire: It refers to the processing heat source using wicker as fuel. There are also willow fires, willow charcoal fires, willow charcoal, and so on.

The charcoal fire: The fire of burning charcoal. Oak charcoal fire is suitable for refining all mineral medicines.

The mulberry fire: One of the traditional processing heat sources. It is a fire formed by the burning of mulberry trees. It is suitable for preparing tonics medicines and boiling all ointments.

The hot ash fire: Also known as hot ash, fire, ash fire. It is the none extinguished fine ashes when burning firewood. It is suitable for " dry by heat" or "roasting" medicines.

稻糠火：指用稻壳作燃料的炮制热源。此火小而缓，炮制药物质量稳定，损耗小，加工量不受限制。常用来煅制石决明、牡蛎，其方法是将稻壳与石决明层层叠放，堆至适宜高度后，点燃稻糠，使其缓缓燃烧至粗糠烧尽。

（2）不同火力、火候：不同的火会有不同的炮制火力和火候，一般可分为武火、中火、文火三种。

武火：为火势猛烈的大火、猛火。饮片气香色艳，与药工擅长武火高温快炒关系颇大，并认为武火一般适宜短时间抢火候快速急炒、蒸制及矿物类药煅制。常用武火快炒的有体重、质实、片大、片厚或对色泽要求高的药材，采用的方法有炒黄、炒焦、炒爆。须用武火炒制的，若火力过弱则饮片色不艳、香不浓；蒸制火力不足则不上大气，蒸药不过心，或者蒸制后切出的饮片色黯、少光泽；无武火则矿物类药煅不透。

中火：为火势和缓的火。炆制、煨制用的大堆糠火亦属中火范围。中火适宜较长时间清炒、炆制、煨制及贝壳类药煅制。如用中火炮制果实种子类或体质松泡、片小或薄的药材，常用于微炒、炒黄和炒爆；也用于滋补药物的炆制、附子等药的煨制。须中火炒的，若火力过猛，则炒制品色泽深暗，甚则焦化、炭化；炆制品火猛则水干药焦；煨制品过火则炭化、灰化。

文火：为比中火火力还小、火焰不旺的微弱火力。是适宜烘焙干燥或蜜炙和熬制至一定程度时转用的维持火力。须用文火炙熬者，火力过大则炙物焦枯、熬胶老化。

The rice bran fire: The rice bran is considered as the heating fuel when processing. This fire is small and gentle, the quality of processing drugs with this fire would be with stable high quality and little effect losing. The processing capacity is not limited. It is often used to calcine the shell of Haliotidis Concha (Shijueming) and Ostreae Concha (Muli). The method is to stack rice bran and Abalone layer by layer, stack to the appropriate height, and ignite rice bran until it slowly burns up.

(2) Different firepower: In addition, all kinds of fire have different firepower, duration, and degree of heating when processing. It is normally divided into high heating, medium heating, and low heating.

The high heating: It is a fierce fire. The fragrance and bright color of the decoction pieces are closely related to the pharmacist's excellence in high-temperature and quick-frying with high heating. It is considered that high heating is suitable for quick stir-frying, steaming, and calcination of mineral drugs in a short time. The suitable herbal medicines include heavy, hard texture, big and thick slices which maybe also need high-quality color demand. The commonly processing methods with high heating include stir-frying to yellow, stir-frying to coke, and stir-frying to the explosion. If the herbal medicine slices that need to be stir-fried with high heating are not stir-fried with suitable heating, the slices would not be with bright color and fragrance. If the firepower is insufficient, the water would not penetrate the center of the medicinal materials which are processed with steaming, or the color of the medicines slices would be dim and less lustrous. The mineral drugs can also only be thoroughly calcined with high heating.

Medium heating: It is gentle heating with fire. The Large piles of bran fires during stewing and roasting are in the range of medium heating. Medium heating is suitable for long-time frying, stewing, roasting, and shellfish calcination. For example, processing the fruit and seeds or crunchy, small, or thin pieces of medicinal materials with medium heating. Medium heating is always used in the processing methods of stir-frying on paper, stir-frying to yellow, and stir-frying to the explosion. It is also used for stewing of nourishing drugs, roasting of Aconiti Lateralis Radix Praeparata (Fuzi), and so on. If the fire is too strong, the stir-fried products will be dim in color, coking, and carbonization. If the fire is too strong in stewing, the water would be dry and the slices would become coke. If the fire is too strong in roasting, the processed products would be carbonized and ashed.

Low heating: It is weak heating that is smaller than medium heating with weak firepower. It is suitable for baking, frying, stir-frying, or decocting with honey to keep the firepower. The herbal medicines that need to be processed with low heating would be scorched and gelatinized if firepower is too strong.

炮制过程中火候应用规律是：蜜炙宜先中火后文火；煮制和砂爆、炒焦、炒炭宜先武火后中火；熬制宜先武火后中火，再以文火收胶；花叶类药炒炭宜先中火后文火，各药炒色（色泽要求高）、蒸制、矿物类药煅制则宜武火到底。

四、蒸煮制工具

蒸、煮、熬用的一般为生铁锅、塘锅灶、圆木甑、蒸笼、蒸屉。

1. 圆木甑

有捧甑和扛甑两种。捧甑为小甑，两边有甑耳，方便手捧，适宜蒸制少量药材。扛甑为大甑，四边有甑耳，耳内有孔可穿绳索，方便起坐。

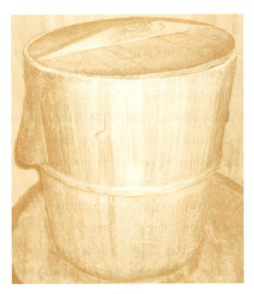

圆木甑

The laws of the heating application are as follows. Using the medium heating first and then the low heating when stir-frying with honey. Using high heating and then medium heating when stir-frying with sand, stir-frying to coke, stir-frying to carbonize. Using high heating and then medium heating and then low heating when decocting. Using medium heating and then low heating when stir-frying flower and leaf medicinal materials to carbonize. Using high heating through the course of processing when stir-frying color medicine materials (with high color requirements), steaming and calcining mineral medicines.

Section Four   Steaming and Boiling Tools

The steaming and boiling tools include a raw iron pan and pond cooking range round wooden Zeng (an ancient earthen utensil for steaming rice), the bamboo steamer, and the steamer tray.

1. The round wooden Zeng

There are two kinds of round wooden Zeng: a holding Zeng and a carrying Zeng. The holding Zeng is a small steamer with an "ears handle" on both sides, which is convenient for holding with both hands. The holding Zeng is an appropriate steamer for steaming medicinal materials in a small amount. The carrying steamer is a big steamer, with "ear handles with holes" on four sides, which is suitable for inserting a rope through the "ear hole" for the convenience of lifting the steamer.

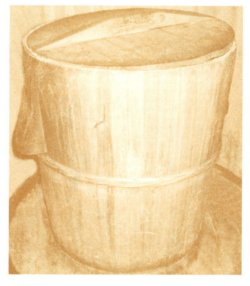

The round wooden Zeng

2. 蒸笼、箅屉

蒸笼为篾制品,圆形、大小不一,一般可设多层。蒸屉为木制品,方屉形、多层。笼屉内均宜垫薄棕网垫。

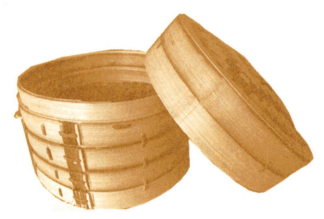

蒸笼、箅屉

五、煅制工具

1. 煅药锅

煅药锅是敞口的铁制煅药锅具。

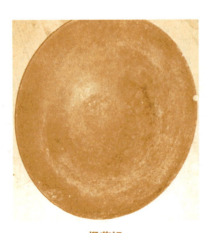

煅药锅

Part II Traditional Processing of Chinese Herbal Medicine

2. The bamboo steamer & the steamer tray

The former is round and woven with a thin bamboo strip. It can be of different sizes with multiple layers. The latter is a square drawer with a multilayer. Inside the drawer, there is a thin palm mat.

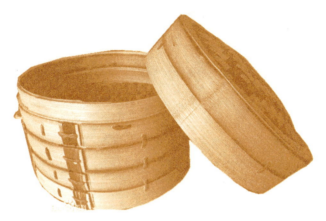

The bamboo steamer & the steamer tray

Section Five   Forging tools

1. The calcining pan

It is an open iron cooker for calcining metal or mineral medicines.

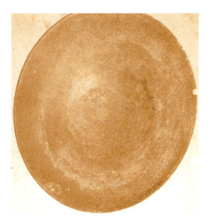

The calcined pan

183

2. 坩埚

坩埚传统为陶土（近代改用耐火泥）制成的无釉容器，专门用来煅制矿物类药物（枯矾除外），置炉灶上或围灶中用，具耐高温、不易破裂的特点。

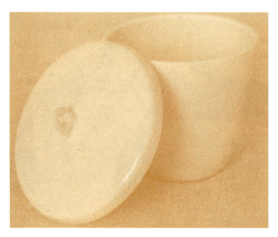

坩埚

3. 阳城罐

此罐俗称嘟噜，为陶制圆筒状罐子，中部膨大，口部与底部略小，为装盛矿石药物隔火坑煅之用，以防止药品过火爆裂粉碎。阳城罐有大小数种，可根据需要选择。

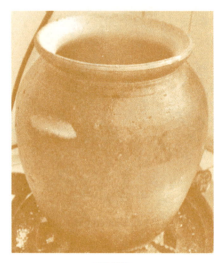

阳城罐

2. The crucible

The traditional crucible is the unglazed container made of clay (modern use refractory mortar), which is dedicated to calcine mineral drugs (except dry alum), and used in the stove or enclosed stove. Its characteristics involve being high temperature resistant and not breaking easily.

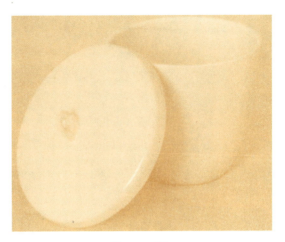

The crucible

3. Yangcheng pot

It is commonly known as "Dulu", a cylindrical container made of ceramic, which has a large central diametrical expansion and a slightly smaller mouth and bottom. It is used for calcining drugs and can prevent the medicine from bursting into pieces. There are several sizes of the Yangcheng pot which can be chosen according to needs.

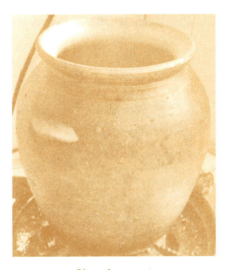

Yangcheng pot

4. 铁汤罐

此为铁制品，上部呈圆筒状，下部较狭，直径 0.5～1 尺，深度 0.8～1.5 尺，适用于煅制容易爆碎的药物。

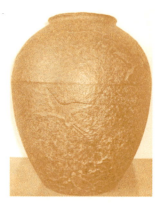

铁汤罐

5. 铁钩

此系铁制细圆杆，前端弯曲，成一双钩，为钩提火煅药罐或翻动药物之用。

6. 炉膛与鼓风器

（1）炉膛：为由炉墙包围起来供燃料燃烧的立体空间。其作用是保证燃料尽可能地燃烧，并使炉膛出口烟气温度冷却到安全工作允许的温度。为此，炉膛应有足够的空间，并布置足够的受热面。此外，应有合理的形状和尺寸，以便于开展炉膛内操作。

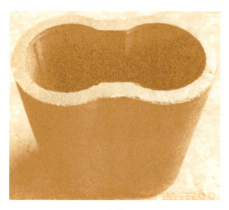

炉膛

4. The iron soup can

It is an iron-made container, the upper part is cylindrical, the lower part is narrow, the diameter is about 15cm ~ 30cm, the depth is 25cm ~ 45cm, it is suitable for calcining drugs easy to the explosion.

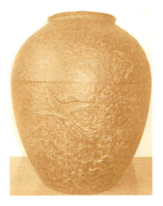

The iron soup can

5. The iron hook

It is a thin round iron rod, its two ends bent to form a double hook shape, and is utilized to lift the calcining pot or simply flip the drugs.

6. Furnace chamber & blower

(1) The furnace chamber: It is a space enclosed by a furnace wall for fuel combustion. Its function is to ensure that the fuel burns as much as possible and cool the venting gas in the furnace to the adequate temperature allowed for safe operation. The furnace chamber should have enough space to get enough heating surface. It should have a reasonable shape and size to operate in the furnace.

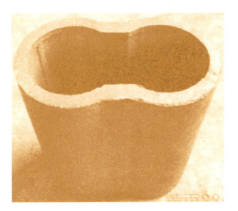

The furnace chamber

（2）鼓风器：包括扇、吹管和皮囊，最早用于强制鼓风的器具是扇和吹管。古埃及金匠曾使用带陶风嘴的吹管，印加人有时用 8～12 根铜管同时吹炼。稍后，发明了用兽皮制作的鼓风皮囊。操作时用绳索拽起皮囊，随后踩下，将风鼓入炉内，以保持煅烧温度。

六、其他制法工具

1. 炆法工具

炆法是将药材润透后，装入陶制炆药坛内加水和辅料，置糠火中用文火慢慢煨煮至熟的制法。常用的工具有炆药坛。炆药坛古称"罂"，即腹大口小的坛子，为无釉陶器（有釉者易烧裂），有耐高温、不易破裂的特点。

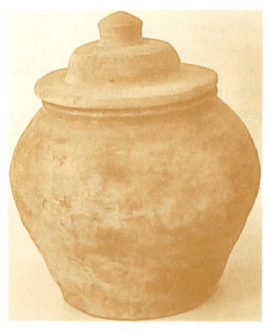

炆药坛

(2) The blower: It has three kinds of instruments: a fan, blowpipe, and leather bag. The earliest instruments used for forcing blowing were a fan and blowpipe. The ancient Egyptian goldsmiths used pipes with earthen mouthpieces, and the Inca sometimes used 8 to 12 brass pipes at one time. Animal skin airbags were invented later. When operating, pulls up leather bag with rope, then step the bag down, the wind would be drummed into the furnace to keep the temperature during calcining.

Section Six Other Tools of Processing

1. The method of stewing

After the medicine is moistened thoroughly, it is placed into the earthen stewing pot with water along with assistant materials. The pot then is placed on the burning chaff with medium heating until the medicine is completely stewed. The commonly used tool is the stewing medicine pot, also known as "Yin" in ancient times, which has a big body and smallmouth, being made of unglazed pottery (the pottery with glaze is easy to crack). The pot is resistant to high temperatures and will not break easily.

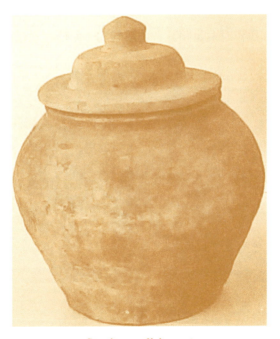

Stewing medicine pot

2. 去油制霜法工具

去油制霜法是药物经过适当加热去油制成松散粉末的方法。常用的工具包括压药板，用于压榨药物去油。

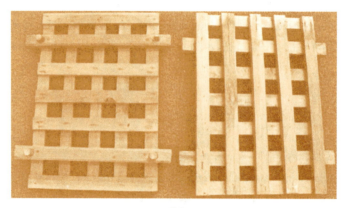

压药板

3. 制绒法工具

制绒法是指某些纤维性和体轻泡的药材经捶打、推碾成绒絮状，可以缓和药性或使药物便于应用，如麻黄碾成绒。常用的工具有铁碾槽，多系生铁铸成，分研槽、研盘两部分，操作时两足踏其上前后转动，使药物通过推研而成绒。

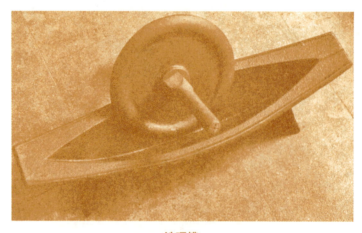

铁碾槽

2. Making frost methods

The main method of making frost is degreasing. It means to make loose powder through heating medicine properly to degrease. The commonly used tool is the pressing plate which can be used for pressing medicines to degrease.

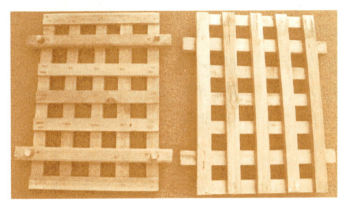

The pressing plate

3. Making fine hair method

It means to pound and press some fibrous and light vesicular herbs into fine hair. The purpose is to moderate the property of medicines and facilitate their application. For example, making Ephedra herba (Mahuang) into fine hair. The commonly used tool is the roller mill groove and pestle which is made of raw iron. Two parts are the grinding mill groove and the roller pestle. When operating, the feet step on the bar to make the pestle move back and forth to make the herbal medicines grind and get fine hair.

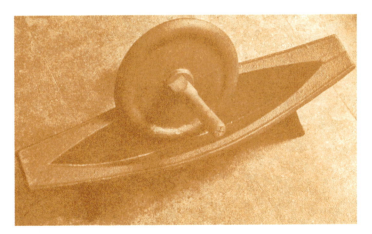

The mill groove and pestle

4. 水飞法工具

某些不溶于水的矿物药,利用粗细粉末在水中悬浮性不同,将不溶于水的矿物、贝壳类药物经反复研磨,而分离制备极细腻粉末的方法,称为水飞法。常用工具有研钵,为瓷制品,外面光滑有釉,内面略粗糙。乳钵棒槌亦为瓷制品,棒槌底下表面粗糙。

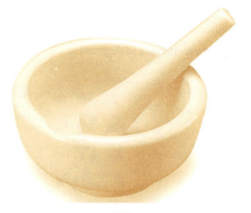

研钵

5. 炼丹工具

火炉是炼丹的重要工具之一,铁、陶、泥质均可。其制法是以一般火炉为基础,然后再在炉子里外搪上一层黄泥,内部的较外部为厚,泥中当混合部分头发、食盐,以免干后开裂,炉膛上小下大,炉口直径或炉膛深度以6寸为合格,炉口须平,以便锅底于炉口密切接合,若全不通气又会削弱炉中火力,故当在炉口左右各开一道缺口以便通气;在火门上方,再开一道直通炉膛的长方形活门,门可开启或关闭,以调节火力。

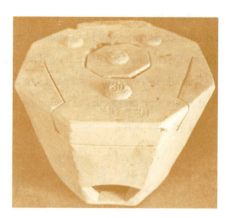

火炉

4. The elutriation

For some mineral drugs that are insoluble in water, the different suspension properties of coarse and fine powder could be used to get fine powder through this method. The insoluble mineral or shell medicines can be ground in water repeatedly to finally get an extremely fine powder. And the method is called 'elutriation'. The commonly used tool is mortar, which is made of porcelain, with a smooth glaze outside and a rough surface inside. And mortar bar is also made of porcelain and has a rough surface.

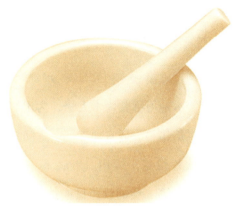

Mortar

5. The alchemy

"The alchemy stove" is one of the most important tools for alchemy, and can be made of iron, pottery, or clay. It is built based on the common stove, a layer of thicker yellow mud is coated all around the stove. The mud in the stove should be sticker than that outside the stove and partially mixed with hair and salt to avoid cracking after drying. The top of the stove is small and large in the below part, with a 20cm diameter of the mouth and depth of the stove. The top of the stove must be flat so the bottom of the pot can be closely connected to the top part of the stove. Without ventilation, the fire

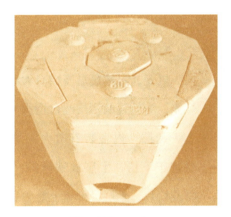

The alchemy stove

in the stove will weaken. There should be an opening gap on the left and right sides of the stove for ventilation. In the upper part of the fire door, there is a door that can open or close to adjust the firepower as needed.

七、干燥工具

1. 烘箱

本地习称其为木火焙,为木制长方形多层烘焙箱箱格,适宜加工厂、车间较大量药材或饮片烘焙干燥用。最底下一层用来遮挡火焰,第二层铺放药材或饮片达16cm厚左右;依次架三层、四层……以达到用适宜温度干燥药材或饮片的目的。

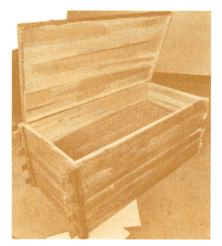

烘箱

2. 烘笼

烘笼,习称篾烘笼,有大篾烘笼和小篾烘笼,为竹篾制两层圆台型火笼,其结构有上下两层,内置装有微火的炉盆火架,上层嵌于下层,上层放铁丝筛,筛上放置药材或饮片。上层顶部盖上篾箩盖(亦称"竹匾"),以保证适宜湿度。适于药店(房)及仓库用炉盆火架烘焙干燥少量饮片及珍贵细料。

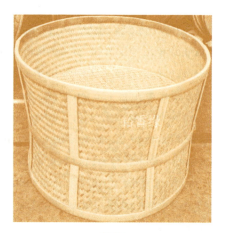

烘笼

Part II Traditional Processing of Chinese Herbal Medicine

Section Seven　Dry tools

1. The oven

Also referred to as a "wooden firebox". It is a multi-layered rectangular wooden baking box, which is suitable for baking and drying a large number of medicinal materials or pieces. The bottom layer is to prevent the flame from burning, the second layer is to place medicine materials or pieces 16cm thick, and then the third layer, the fourth layer, etc. The purpose is to dry the medicine materials or pieces at the appropriate temperature.

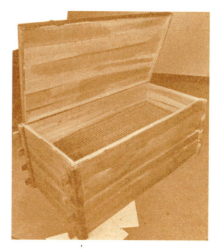

The oven

2. The roaster

Also known as the "bamboo roaster". There are two types of a roaster: big-stripped roaster and small-stripped roaster. It is a two-layer round-table fire cage made of bamboo sticks. The structure is upper and lower layers. Inside it is a brazier with a small fire (covering the ash). The upper layer is embedded in the lower layer. The iron wire sieve is put on the upper layer and the medicine materials or pieces are put on the sieve. The top of the upper layer should be cover with a bamboo cover (also known as the "bamboo plaque") to keep proper humidity. It is suitable for drying a small number of pieces of precious fine materials in drugstores and warehouses.

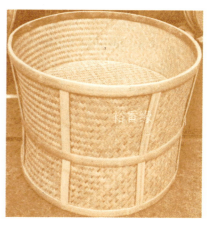

The roaster

3. 烘桶

烘桶呈圆形筒状，直径约 1.8 尺，高约 2.5～3 尺，上无盖，下无底，内可放置风炉燃火，上放置筛子烘药。

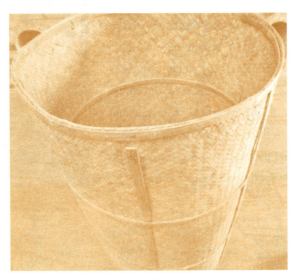

烘桶

3. The baking bucket

It is cylindrical with approximately 35 cm diameter of 80 cm to 1-meter height. There is no cover on the top or bottom. The stove is placed inside and a sieve with medicine materials or pieces on it is placed on the top of the bucket.

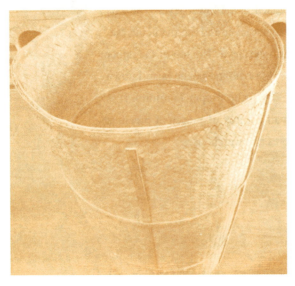

The Baked barrels

参考文献：

[1] 吴文辉，伍淳操，郭小红，等.重庆市传统中药炮制技术传承现状与分析[J].中国医院药学杂志，207，37（19）：1883-1926.

[2] 成莉.宋以前中药炮制文献研究[D].北京：中国中医科学院，2010.

[3] 郑文杰.《本草纲目》中"修治"术语的探讨[D].北京：中国中医科学院，2016.

[4] 刘文凤.试述中药的炮制与临床疗效[J].中医药导报，2011，17（03）：100-101.

[5] 王若晴.龟龄集制药工艺及其保护传承研究[D].太原：山西大学，2013.

[6] 罗伟雄.风选在炮制中的应用[J].中成药，1989（08）：45.

[7] 王琦，孙立立，贾天柱.中药饮片炮制发展回眸[J].中成药，2000（01）：35-60.

[8] 林汉芳.浅谈中药炮制的基本操作[J].中医药研究，2002（06）：20-21.

[9] 谭庆佳.中药炮制工艺改进[N].中国中医药报，2002-03-21.

[10] 白棠.王德吉力虎.蒙药与中药炮制的不同[J].世界最新医学信息文摘,2018,18(63):182.

[11] 张怀清.中药炮制对临床疗效的影响[J].内蒙古中医药,2013,32(06):83-84.

[12] 赖中福,杨绍合.浅述砻糠在煅法炮制中的应用[J].中国药业,2003(08):56-57.

[13] 张金莲,谢日健,罗文华,等.建昌帮特色辅料"糠"应用形式及其与药共制的作用[J].江西中医药大学学报,2016,28(02):57-58+67.

[14] 裴艳秋,颜霞.对中药净选作用的认识[J].黑龙江中医药,2001(05):54-56.

[15] 张凤玲.论中药炮制的方法[J].北方药学,2015,12(09):120-121.

[16] 辛二旦,司昕蕾,边甜甜,等.大黄产地趁鲜切制工艺优选及与传统加工的比较研究[J].时珍国医国药,2020,31(06):1368-1370.

[17] 马柏森.谈中药饮片的加工[J].中药通报,1983(05):41-45.

[18] 包献珍.中药巨匠朱清山第十二章有序传承[J].时代报告(奔流),2020(02):140-157.

[19] 邱玏,朱建平.道教外丹术对《雷公炮炙论》的影响[J].江西中医学院学报,2005(02):21-23.

[20] 杨冬生.润法在中药炮制中的应用[J].江西中医药,1995(S3):95.

[21] 吴珊珊，何席呈，王建科，等.中药炮制传统技术实训模式改革探索[J].中国中医药现代远程教育，2019，17（12）：137-139.

[22] 关怀，王地，王敏，等.古代中药炮制学史分期考[J].北京中医药，2009，28（08）：629-631.

[23] 房志雄.传统中药炮制技艺之切制饮片——老药工可用手工刀将一个槟榔切成108片[J].首都食品与医药，2016，23（05）：58-59.

[24] 宋丽丽.不同区域中药炮制特色技术探讨[J].临床医药文献电子杂志，2020，7（34）：191.

[25] 杨冰，蔡宝昌，张洪雷.江西省中药文化软实力[J].江西科学，2017，35（02）：318-322.

[26] 原思通.知药须先懂医 治学当勤积累[N].中国中医药报，2011-09-07（003）.

[27] 李红伟，田连起，李娴，等.不同地域中药炮制特色技术研究[J].中国中医药现代远程教育，2017，15（02）：42-43.

[28] 陈宏伟.中药特色技术的起承转合[J].中国中医药现代远程教育，2018，16（14）：155-158.

[29] 黄秋云，潘鸿贞，赵蕾.福州市中药炮制历史和现状调研[J].海峡药学，2009，21（11）：254-255.

[30] 张博华，张义生.竹茹炮制研究进展[J].湖北中医杂志，2013，35（10）：76-79.

［31］周逸群，李瑞，贺玉婷，等．中药"炒炭存性"炮制共性技术的研究现状及超分子"印迹模板"表征技术的提出［J］．中国中药杂志，2019，44（19）：4293-4299．

［32］张金莲，曾昭君，潘旭兰，等．砻糠在建昌帮中药炮制中的应用［J］．中草药，2013，44（21）：3092-3094．

［33］钟凌云，龚千锋，杨明，等．传统炮制技术流派特点及发展［J］．中国中药杂志，2013，38（19）：3405-3408．

［34］贾春华，庄享静．烹饪技术移植后萌发的中药炮制理论［J］．中国科学：生命科学，2016，46（08）：1008-1014．

［35］孟江，张英，曹晖，等．岭南中药炮制特色探析［J］．中国实验方剂学杂志，2020，26（06）：193-200．

［36］祁晓鸣，孟祥龙，何美菁，王等．生地黄制炭（炒炭、煅炭）前后凉血止血作用比较研究［J］．中国中药杂志，2019，44（05）：954-961．

［37］孟祥龙，马俊楠，崔楠楠，等．基于热分析的炉甘石煅制研究［J］．中国中药杂志，2013，38（24）：4303-4308．

［38］陈云，陈劲松，郁红礼，等．胆南星发酵制品与混合蒸制品的鉴别研

究[J].世界中医药,2019,14(02).

[39] 吴晓东,林楠,陈华师.蒸制陈皮炮制工艺的研究[J].中国药师,2011,14(09):1265-1267.

[40] 常慧芳.探讨中药炮制中炒、炙、煅、蒸、煮与疗效的关系[J].世界最新医学信息文摘,2017,17(01):124+126.

[41] 胡律江,胡志方,王小平,等.江西建昌帮炆熟地黄的HPLC指纹图谱[J].中国实验方剂学杂志,2015,21(23):33-36.

[42] 易炳学,钟凌云,龚千锋.江西建昌帮炆法特色炮制及其现代研究思路[J].时珍国医国药,2012,23(07):1755-1756.

[43] 霍韬光,郭婧潭,张颖花,等.水飞法炮制对雄黄中可溶性硫和砷含量的影响[J].辽宁中医杂志,2016,43(02):360-361.

[44] 李超英,滕利荣,魏秀德,等.朱砂水飞炮制工艺及质量标准研究[J].中成药,2008,30(12):1806-1809.

[45] 李超英,魏秀德,王凯,等.雄黄水飞炮制工艺及其机制研究[J].中国药房,2008(27):2151-2153.

Part III
第三部分

现代研究
Modern Research of PCHM

第五章 炮制的现代研究概况

一、概述

1. 中药炮制研究的意义

中药炮制经过长期发展,已经形成了以中医药理论为指导的完整体系,利用现代科技手段,对中药炮制已经进行了许多深入的研究,取得了一定的成果,但目前还存在许多不足。因此,进一步开展中药炮制的深入系统研究,对中药炮制学科、产业的发展具有重要意义。

通过中药炮制研究,可为中药炮制原理、技术方法提供科技支撑,利于传承中药炮制经验和保护非物质文化遗产。中国历代医学家在长期的医疗实践中,不断总结积累制药经验,逐渐形成了独具特色的理论,中药炮制技术已列入国家级非物质文化遗产。全国各地积累的炮制经验总结研究已基本上完成了汇总,开展了较系统的文献研究,对常用中药饮片的炮制原理、工艺、设备及标准等进行了相应研究,取得了一定的成绩。但研究的深度和广度不够,能阐明中药炮制原理的品种少,研究成果得到推广应用的更少。因此,应强调运用化学、药理、生物、信息等多学科的现代技术方法研究,扩大研究的品种范围,为阐明中药炮制的科学内涵、规范工艺及制定参数、拟订质量标准提供科学依据,以利于炮制技术的传承和保护。

第三部分 现代研究

Part III Modern Research of PCHM

Chapter Five   The Introduction of Modern Research of PCHM

Section One   The Summary

1. Significance of research on PCHM

After a long period of development, PCHM has formed a complete system guided by TCM theory. Much in-depth research has been done by utilizing modern scientific and technological methods, and some achievements have been made. However, there are still many deficiencies at present, so it will be of great significance to do systematic research on PCHM, which is beneficial to the development of the subject and industry of PCHM.

The research on the PCHM can provide scientific and technological support for the principle and technology, which facilitates to inherit and protect the experience of the PCHM belonging to intangible cultural heritage. In the long-term medical practice of history, Chinese medical experts have summarized and accumulated pharmaceutical experience and gradually formed unique theories. Besides, the processing technology of traditional Chinese medicine has been listed in the national intangible cultural heritage of China. The research on processing experience accumulated in different parts of the country has been collected throughout the country, and systematic literature studies have been carried out. However, the depth and ranges of the research are not enough, and the herbal medicines that can clarify the principle of PCHM are few, and the research results are less widely used either. Therefore, it is necessary to emphasize the application of modern technology and methods, expanding the scope of research by using the knowledge of chemistry, pharmacology, biology, information, and other subjects, to expand the range of studies of herbal medicines, clarify the PCHM principles, standardize the PCHM technology, formulate parameters of PCHM technology, as well as the quality standards of herbal medicines slices or pieces, to facilitate the inheritance and protection of PCHM.

通过中药炮制研究，发展创新中药炮制理论与炮制技术方法有利于提高行业整体水平。如何在继承的基础上，运用现代科学技术研究成果，以新的思维和观点，创新与发展炮制理论和技术方法，是中药炮制学科必须重视的问题。研究要有突出中药炮制特点的思维、设计和评价等，吸收最新的科技成果，借鉴中药相关学科研究技术手段，创新中药炮制理论，发展炮制技术方法，提高研究水平，加快研究成果的应用，从而提高行业整体技术水平，为促进中药炮制的现代化、国际化发展奠定坚实的研究基础。

2. 中药炮制研究的指导思想

（1）**以中医药理论为指导**：不同的研究内容只有结合相关的中医药理论，才能使研究工作既保持和突出中医药特色，又可揭示其现代科学本质内涵。中医药理论核心和特色最根本的是整体观、辨证论治和综合作用。中医把人体视为一个有机的整体，并把人体与外界环境也视为一个有机整体，把疾病视为病因作用于人体整体反应，诊断和治疗时将人体和疾病置于系统之中统筹考虑。中药本身也是一个系统，其中存在着多种化学成分，主要有二类：一类是有机化合物；一类是无机化合物。各种成分间的相互作用和影响十分复杂。一种或几种化学成分单体，往往不能代表中药的物质基础。中医用药绝不只是用单体成分，例如，黄连和黄柏中皆含小檗碱，但黄连与黄柏并不能相互替代使用。因此，中药炮制研究如果脱离了中医药理论和中医临床用药经验的指导，仅从单一成分（有时仅是指标成分）或适合纯化学成分的某种药理实验来研究和评价中药炮制作用是不够完善的。再如，苦杏仁制霜药用，如果过于强调除尽脂肪油，则有悖于中医传统理论及临床用药原则。中医认为：咳喘属肺，肺与大肠相表里，临床见有痰浊壅塞、肺气不宣的喘满，往往兼有便秘或下痢等症，治疗时宣通肺气，则大便自调；反之，大便秘结，也可引起气肺气喘满，治疗时使大便通畅，则喘满亦可消失。因此，如果单纯从止咳平喘作用出发，仅考虑保存苦杏仁苷，而榨去润肠作用的苦杏仁油，忽视苦杏仁在临床上的整体治疗作用，则难以达到理想疗效。苦杏仁中的苦杏仁苷有镇咳平喘作用，而百里香素则有明显的祛痰作用，所以口服苦杏仁煎剂后，有镇咳、祛痰两种效果，如果单用苦杏仁苷对苦杏仁的功效作微观化解释显然是不全面的。

Through the research of PCHM, developing and innovating PCHM theory and processing technology is beneficial to improve the overall level of the PCHM industry. How to apply modern scientific technology and research findings to innovate and develop the theories and technologies with new ideas based on inheritance is the necessary key problem of PCHM. The research of PCHM should include the thinking, design, and evaluation with PCHM characteristics use the latest scientific and technological achievements of related disciplines of TCM to innovate theory of PCHM, develop the processing technology and methods, improve the research level, speed up the application of research results, thereby to enhance the whole technical level of the industry, to provide a solid foundation for promoting the modernization and internationalization of TCM.

2. Guiding ideology of PCHM research

(1) Guided by the theory of TCM: Only by combining the researches with relevant theories of TCM can the research work keep the characteristics of TCM and clarify the scientific connotation either. The core and characteristics of TCM theory are the whole views, the dialectical treatment, and the comprehensive function. In TCM the human body is regarded as an organic whole, and the human body and the external environment are as an organic whole too. The disease is considered as the etiology acting on the overall response of the body, and the body and the disease are put into the system for overall consideration when diagnosing and treating. For Chinese herbal medicine, it is also a system, in which there are many chemical components, which can be divided into two types: one is organic compounds and another is inorganic compounds. The interaction and influence of various components are very complex. One or several components often do not represent the material basis of Chinese herbal medicine. It is not only used monomer ingredients for treatment in TCM clinic, for example, Berberine contained in both Goptidis Rhizoma (Huanglian) and Phellodendri Chinensis Cortex (Huangbai), but they can not be replaced each other. Therefore, it is not perfect to study and evaluate the effect of PCHM only from a single component (sometimes only index component) or some pharmacological experiment which is only suitable for the pure chemical component if the research on PCHM is separated from the guidance of TCM theory and clinical experience. For example, when making Armeniacae Semen Amarum (Kuxingren) to frost, if putting too much emphasis on the degrease, it will be contrary to the traditional theory of TCM and clinical principles. In TCM, it is thought that cough and asthma are induced from the lung channel, and the lung and the large intestine being interior-exteriorly related, the phlegm obstruction and obstruction of pulmonary qi in asthmatic cough are always combining with constipation or dysentery in the clinic. When treating, promote lung qi, defecate self-adjustment, conversely, the big constipation knot can also cause lung qi asthma full, the good bowel movements will lead to the disappear of asthma. Therefore, it is difficult to achieve the ideal therapeutic effect if we only consider the preservation of amygdalin to relieve cough and asthma, while removing the oil of amygdalas with moistening intestine action, which would ignore the overall therapeutic effect of Armeniacae Semen Amarum (Kuxingren) in clinical practice. The amygdalin in Armeniacae Semen Amarum (Kuxingren) has the effect of relieving cough and asthma, cymene has the obvious effect of reducing phlegm, so after oral administration of Armeniacae Semen Amarum (Kuxingren) decoction, the effect showed relieving cough and reducing phlegm. It is not comprehensive to explain the effect of Armeniacae Semen Amarum (Kuxingren) if only with amygdalin.

（2）以现代科学技术为手段：强调以中医药理论为指导并非否定运用现代医药知识和手段。近年来，已广泛应用化学、药理学、微生物学、免疫学、生物化学、物理学等科学技术，对中药炮制的原理、方法、工艺等方面进行了部分研究，取得了较多的成果。例如，借助化学和药理学技术，已基本阐明乌头类中药的毒性成分和炮制降低其毒性的机制。乌头中含多种生物碱，其中以双酯型的乌头碱毒性最强。乌头药材经加水、加热处理，使双酯型乌头碱第 8 位碳原子上的乙酰基水解（或分解），失去一分子醋酸，得到相应的苯甲酰单酯型乌头次碱类，其毒性为双酯型乌头碱的 $1/200 \sim 1/500$；再进一步是第 14 位碳原子上的苯甲酰基水解（或分解），失去一分子苯甲酸，得到亲水性氨基醇型乌头原碱类，其毒性仅为双酯型乌头碱的 $1/2000 \sim 1/4000$。此外，乌头炮制减毒的另一个原因还可能是炮制过程中脂肪酰基取代了第 8 位碳原子上的乙酰基，生成毒性较低的酯碱之故。乌头炮制过程中，毒性降低的程度，取决于双酯型乌头碱的分解程度，与其总生物碱量无关。

二、中药炮制研究的内容

1. 传统经验与历史文献的研究

要研究中药炮制，首先要了解炮制的现状。中华人民共和国成立后，在调查和总结传统炮制经验方面做了大量工作，陆续整理出版了各省、市《中药饮片炮制规范》和《中药炮制经验集成》，近年来又相继出版了《中药饮片炮制述要》《中药临床生用与制用》《新编中药炮制法》《樟树中药炮制全书》《中药炮制与临床应用》《中药炮制学》等，为中药炮制的生产、教学、科研提供了重要参考。

(2) Utilizing modern science and technology: To emphasize the guiding of TCM theory doesn't mean to deny modern scientific knowledge and technology. In recent years, chemistry, pharmacology, microbiology, immunology, biochemistry, physics, and other scientific technologies have been widely used in researches on the principles, methods, and techniques of the PCHM and achieved many results. For example, with the help of chemical and pharmacological techniques, the toxic components of aconite herbs and the mechanism of processing to reduce their toxicity have been clarified. Aconite contains many alkaloids, among which the diester-type aconite is the most toxic. The acetyl group on the 8th carbon atom of diester type aconitine was hydrolyzed (or decomposed) and one molecule of acetic acid was lost. Furthermore, the benzoyl group on the 14th carbon atom was hydrolyzed (or decomposed), one molecule of benzoic acid was lost and forms hydrophilic amino alcohol type aconitine whose toxicity is only 1/2000 ~ 1/4000 of that of diester type aconitine. In addition, another reason for reducing toxicity in processing aconite may be that the fatty acyl group replaces the acetyl group on the 8th carbon atom during processing, resulting in an ester base with less toxicity. The degree of toxicity reduction during the processing of aconite depends on the decomposition degree of diester-type aconitine and has no relation to the total alkaloid content.

Section Two   Research on the PCHM

1. Research on traditional experience and historical documents

To study the PCHM, the status of PCHM should be understood first. After the founding of the People's Republic of China (PRC), a lot of investigating and summarizing of the traditional processing experience has been done, *Chinese Medicine Yinpian Concocted Norms* (*Zhongyao Yinpian Paozhi Guifan*) and *Processing Experience Integration* (*Zhongyao Paozhi Jingyan Jicheng*) have been edited and published. In recent years, *The Review of Processing of Chinese Herbal Medicine* (*Zhongyao Paozhi Shuyao*), *Application of Raw and Processed Chinese Herbal Medicine in TCM Clinical* (*Zhongyao Linchuang Shengyong yu Zhiyong*), *Newly compiled Processing of Chinese Herbal Medicine methods* (*Xinbian Zhongyao Paozhifa*), Book of Processing of Chinese Herbal Medicine in Zhangshu"(*Zhangshu Zhongyao Paozhi Quanshu*), *Processing of Chinese Herbal Medicine and Clinical Application* (*Zhongyao Paozhi yu Linchuang Yingyong*), *Processing of Chinese Herbal Medicine* (*Zhongyao Paozhixue*) has been published, which provide an important reference for the production, teaching, and studying of PCHM.

研究中药炮制除了研究传统炮制经验外，还必须搞清炮制的历史沿革，系统整理相关历史文献。中国中医科学院中药研究所等单位摘录汉代至清代167部古代中医药书籍中有关炮制内容，出版了《历代中药炮制资料辑要》，对研究炮制的起源、原始意图和演变过程提供了部分历史资料。王孝涛研究员等又在此基础上，编辑出版了《历代中药炮制法汇典》，分古代和现代二册。古代部分搜集常用中药清代以前（包括清代）的主要炮制文献，每味药按处方用名、炮制方法、炮制作用系统整理；现代部分以收集《中国药典》和全国各地中药饮片炮制规范资料为基础，增添了1985年以前有关现代科研技术资料等内容，每味药按来源、炮制方法、现代研究系统整理。全书共收载常用中药552种，为中医药教学、科研、临床及生产提供了丰富的文献资料。

2. 炮制理论与炮制原理研究

中药炮制理论与中医药理论密不可分，是中医中药人员在漫长的用药实践中总结而成的，是中医药学理论体系的重要组成部分。中药炮制理论包括中药制药（原则和制法）理论、中药生熟理论、辅料作用理论和药性变化理论。例如，将中药炮制原则归纳为：相反为制，相资为制，相畏为制，相恶为制。将辅料制药归纳为：酒制升提，姜制发散，入盐走肾脏仍仗软坚，用醋注肝经且资住痛等。通过现代研究探讨炮制理论的科学内涵，不但有利于炮制原理的阐述，而且将指导炮制方法的改革与创新。

第三部分 现代研究
Part III Modern Research of PCHM

In addition to studying the traditional processing experience, the research on the PCHM must also make clear the historical evolution of the processing and systematically sort out relevant historical documents. The Institute of Chinese Materia Medica and other institutions of the Chinese Academy of Traditional Chinese Medicine extracted the contents related to the processing of 167 ancient Chinese medicine books from the Han Dynasty to the Qing Dynasty, and published *The compilation of PCHM Data of All Dynasties* (*Lidai Zhongyao Paozhi Ziliao Jiyao*), providing some historical data on the origin, original intention, and evolution of PCHM. Based on this, Pro. Wang Xiaotao has edited and published the *PCHM Methods in Ancient Books* (*Lidai Paozhifa Huidian*) which includes two parts of ancient and modern time. The ancient part collected the PCHM methods record is commonly used TCM books before the Qing Dynasty (including the Qing Dynasty), the prescription, processing methods, and processing effect of each herbal medicine were recorded. In the modern part, there collected the contents of *Chinese Pharmacopoeia*, the Processing Specifications across the country, and the study results of PCHM before 1985. The resource, processing methods, and studies of PCHM of each herbal medicine were systematically organized There are 552 kinds of commonly used traditional Chinese herbal medicines in the book, providing a wealth of literature for the teaching, researching, clinical, and production of TCM.

2. Research on processing theory and principle

The theory of PCHM is closely related to the theory of TCM, which is summarized by TCM personnel in the long practice of TCM use and is an important part of the theoretical system of TCM. The theory of PCHM includes the theory of pharmacy (principle and processing methods) of TCM, the theory of raw and processed products of traditional Chinese herbal medicines, the theory of assistant material processing action, and the theory of property change PCHM. For example, the principles of PCHM were summarized as, processing with assistant materials with opposite nature, processing with assistant materials with same nature, processing to reduce side effects, and processing to reduce toxicity. The theories of assistant materials processing effects were summarized as, promoting the effect of medicines through processing with wine, enhancing the effect of dispelling after processing with ginger, inducing to affect the kidney channel after processing with salt, inducing to affect the liver channel to ease the pain after processing with vinegar, etc. To discuss the scientific connotation of processing theories through modern research will not only help to clarify the processing mechanism but also to guide the reform and innovation of processing methods.

中药炮制原理的研究就是探讨中药炮制减毒、增效、缓性或产生新药效的机制，这是炮制研究的核心。只有了解中药炮制前后理化性质和药理作用的变化，以及这些变化的临床意义，才能对炮制方法作出较科学的评价，指导和促进炮制方法的改进，制订饮片质量标准，提高药品质量，确保临床用药有效安全。目前已有的研究多集中于有毒中药的炮制、传统认为炮制前后作用差异较大的品种、炭药，以及药材已知成分和药理作用与中医所说的药效接近的品种。不少研究成果对阐明中药炮制的科学内涵和临床用药理论具有重要的意义。

3. 炮制方法与工艺研究

由于历史的原因，目前各地中药炮制仍存在一药多法、各地各法的现象，要采用现代科学技术，对一种中药的不同炮制方法进行比较，探明不同炮制方法对中药物质基础、药理作用和临床疗效的影响，以综合评价不同炮制方法的合理性和可行性，从而淘汰落后的、不合理的炮制方法，建立科学合理的适于现代化生产的炮制方法。炮制方法明确后、应进一步筛选和优化炮制工艺，应对炮制工艺的各个因素进行考察，规范炮制工艺技术参数，技术参数应包括传统经验的主观指标，也包括现代的客观指标，两者相结合的技术参数使炮制工艺具有简便、实用可行的特点。

炮制工艺的改革和创新也是中药炮制研究的重要内容之一，在炮制原理明确的基础上，对原有炮制工艺进行改进或创新。如草乌传统炮制多采用浸泡、水煮制或蒸制的方法，在其炮制降毒机制明确的基础上，提出采用"高压蒸制"的炮制改进方法。炮制工艺改革和创新的目的是提高生产效率，降低生产成本，保证临床安全有效。改进炮制方法和工艺是中药炮制研究的长期任务和重要内容。

The research on the principle of PCHM is to explore the PCHM mechanism of reducing toxicity, increasing effect, moderating properties, or producing new effects. which is the core of the processing research. Only by understanding the changes of physical and chemical properties and pharmacological effects before and after the PCHM, as well as the clinical significance of these changes, can we make a more scientific evaluation of the processing methods, guide and promote the improvement of the processing methods, formulate the quality standards for decoction pieces, improve the quality of drugs, and ensure the effective and safe clinical use. Nowadays the existing researches of PCHM mainly focus on the processing of toxic herbal medicines, or those being traditionally considered to have great differences in effects before and after processing, or charcoal medicines, or those whose components and pharmacological effects are already known close to the effects of TCM. Many research results had great significance to elucidate the scientific connotation and clinical medication theory of PCHM.

3. Research on processing method and technology

For historical reasons, there still exists the phenomenon that one herbal medicine processed with multiple methods or processing one herbal medicine with different methods in different places, which need to explore the influence on the material base, pharmacological action, and clinical curative effect through different processing methods, to comprehensively evaluate the rationality and feasibility of different processing methods. Only by doing so, the unreasonable processing methods could be discarded and the scientific and reasonable modern processing methods being suitable for production could be established. After making clear the processing method, the processing technologies could be further screened out and optimized, the parameters of processing technology could be inspected and standardized. The technical parameters of processing technology include the subjective indicators of traditional experience, as well as the modern objective indicators. The parameters with two aspects have the characteristics of simple, practical and feasible.

The reform and innovation of the processing techniques are also one of the important contents of the research of PCHM. For example, the traditional processing of Aconiti Kusnezoffii Radix (Caowu) is mostly by soaking, boiling, or steaming. Based on the clear mechanism of its processing, the improvement method of "high-pressure steaming" is put forward. The aim of the reform and innovation of processing technology is to improve production efficiency, reduce production cost, and ensure clinical safety and effectiveness. It is a long-term task and important content to improve the processing method and technology of PCHM.

4. 饮片质量标准研究

饮片质量标准是控制药品质量，保证临床用药有效安全的重要内容。而科学的炮制理论和工艺是确保饮片质量的前提条件。评价一个药物的质量应包括三个方面，即真实性、纯度和品质优良度。真实性是通过药物来源、性状和鉴别项目来体现的，纯度是通过有关检查项目来测定的，品质优良度是由浸出物含量和有效成分的含量测定来予以衡量的。国家有关部门现在很重视饮片质量标准的研究工作，《中国药典》1995年版开始对有些中药饮片规定总灰分、酸不溶性灰分等指标的最高限量值。今后饮片质量标准的研究必须将经验鉴别与现代方法和手段紧密结合，可以从炮制品性状、净度、水分、灰分、浸出物量、有效成分和有毒成分的含量等方面加以研究，并注重饮片专属性质量标准的相关研究。

4. Study on the quality standards of prepared slices

The quality standard of decoction pieces is an important content to control the quality of drugs and ensure effective and safe clinical use. And scientific processing theory and technology is the prerequisite to ensure the quality of prepared slices. Evaluation of the quality of a drug should include three aspects: authenticity, purity, and quality. Authenticity is reflected by the source, character, and identification items of the drug, purity is determined by the relevant inspection index, and quality is decided by the content of the extract and active ingredients. The quality standard of decoction pieces is now taken seriously by the relevant departments of the state. The maximum limits of the total ash content and acid insoluble ash content of some TCM decoction pieces have been stipulated since the 1995 edition of *Chinese pharmacopeia*. In the future, the study on the quality standard of decoction pieces must combine the empirical identification with modern methods and means, and it can be studied from the aspects of the characteristics of processed products, purity, moisture, ash content, extract quantity, active ingredients, and toxic ingredients, and much more attention should be paid on the study on the exclusive quality standards of decoction pieces.

5. 辅料质量标准的研究

用辅料炮制中药是传统制药的一大特色。炮制辅料按照形态分为液体辅料和固体辅料，液体辅料主要包括酒、醋、蜂蜜、食盐水、生姜汁、甘草汁、黑豆汁、胆汁、吴茱萸汁等，其中以酒、醋、盐、姜、蜜应用最多，固体辅料主要包括大米、蛤粉、滑石粉、油砂、麦麸、白矾、豆腐等。现代对辅料炮制的研究大多是研究改进辅料炮制工艺和（或）辅料炮制对药效的影响，而对辅料本身的研究较少。因炮制辅料质量的优劣直接影响饮片质量和临床疗效，故其规范化、标准化是亟待解决的问题。2004年国家启动了炮制辅料规范化的研究，针对炮制辅料的品质、规格、工艺、质量标准等方面进行了初步研究和探索。"十五"期间又启动了"酒醋炮制辅料示范性研究"，科技部公益性研究工作又资助了"食药两用8种炮制辅料药用标准研究"。迄今为止，已对约10种炮制辅料进行了立项研究，这些研究将对中药饮片炮制实施质量监督管理起到重要作用。但是，由于不同辅料品种质量标准的基础研究工作并不平衡，有的已有较完善的药用标准（如滑石）；有的已有食品国家标准（如酒、醋、蜜、盐等）。有的仅有其他行业的标准；有相当一部分没有标准。因此，应根据辅料品种质量标准的现状设计研究方案，对已有标准的可以借鉴并开展进一步研究，增加或调整炮制辅料特定的质量控制项目，以此完善提高标准，如调整食醋总酸的规定量、增加薄层鉴别等；仅有其他行业标准的，借鉴此类标准应慎重，应特别关注其安全性指标的研究；尚无任何质量标准的，应结合辅料生产实际和炮制应用情况，对其质量标准进行系统研究，建立符合药用要求的质量标准。

5. Research on quality standards of assistant materials

Using assistant materials to process traditional Chinese herbal medicines is one of the characteristics of TCM. The processing assistant materials can be divided into liquid and solid materials, liquid materials mainly include wine, vinegar, honey, salt water, ginger, Glycyrrhizae Radix Et Rhizoma juice, black soybean juice, bile, Evodia rutaecarpa juice, etc., among them the wine, cool, salt, ginger, honey are commonly used. Most solid materials including rice, clam powder, talcum powder, oil sands, wheat bran, alum, tofu, etc. Modern research of processing assistant materials is mostly about improving processing technology with assistant materials or studying the influence on herbal medicines' pharmaceutical effect, less on assistant materials themselves. Since the quality of assistant materials affects the decoction pieces and clinical effects directly, the normalization and standardization of assistant materials are urgent problems that need to be solved. In 2004, the state initiated the research on the standardization of processing assistant materials, the preliminary research and exploration have been done on quality, specification, technology, and quality standard of assistant materials. During the tenth five-year plan period, "Demonstration research on processing assistant materials of wine and vinegar" has been done, and the public welfare research work of the ministry of science and technology also funded "Research on the medical standards for 8 processing assistant materials for both food and medicine". So far, about 10 kinds of processing assistant materials have been studied, which will play an important role in the quality supervision and management of the PCHM. However, due to the imbalance of basic research work on quality standards of different kinds of assistant materials, some assistant materials have built better standards (such as talc), some have food national standards (such as wine, vinegar, honey, salt, etc.) And some only have other industries standard. Quite a few have no standards. Therefore, research programs should be designed according to the current situation of quality standards of assistant materials, and further studies should be conducted to improve the existing quality standards of assistant materials adding or adjusting specific quality control index to improve the standard, such as adjusting the prescribed amount of total acid of vinegar, increasing the identification of thin layer, etc. Only with other industry standards, it should be careful to reference such standards and pay special attention to its safety indicators. If there is no quality standard yet, the quality standard should be systematically studied according to the actual production and processing application of the assistant materials to establish the quality standard that meets medical requirements.

6. 中药加工炮制设备的研究

中药加工炮制生产长期以来主要靠手工操作，生产规模小，个体差异大，饮片质量难以控制。因此，为实现中药饮片生产的规范化和规模化，开展炮制设备研究也是炮制研究的一个重要内容。

20 世纪 60 年代以后逐步引用或研制了一些机械设备。

在净制方面，近年来不断采用多种电动机械代替手工操作。在洗药设备方面，目前主要有滚筒式、刮板式、链板式等几种类型洗药机。在药材软化工序方面，有减压冷浸软化装置，既可使药材达到软化要求，又可保证饮片质量，提高工效约 30 倍。用多功能提取罐加压快速引润法或真空喷气快速引润法，可大大缩短药材软化时间，保证饮片质量。在切药设备方面，主要有剁刀式和旋转式中药切药机。

在炒制设备方面，滚筒式炒药机上加一个简单的喷头装置，就可用于须边炒边喷洒液体辅料药材的炮制；对转鼓式炒药机改装 3 个不同转速调速器，可基本满足各类中药炮制时的温度要求，如不同型号的炒药机、红外线中药炒药机、电热式炒药机、电子程控炒药机和中药电脑炒药机等。电子程控炒药机采用顺序控制器，使投料、炒药、出料、过筛、风选、吹冷、包装均能自动操作。中药电脑炒药机采用电子计算机终端控制系统，具有烘烤加温、恒温、程序升温功能，由计算机输入各项炒药工艺参数，实现自动开门进料、自动控制搅拌的转速和开停自动定量喷淋液体辅料、自动排烟排气、自动开门出料。装有工艺记录仪表，可进行工艺数据的储存和录制，工艺数据和工作状况还可在终端屏幕汉字显示，并以汉字问答式输入操作。发生机械故障时有电器保护和报警装置，备有自动和手动两套工艺控制系统。该机适用于药物的多种加工炮制。

在饮片干燥方面，常用的有翻板式干燥机、热风干燥机、远红外辐射干燥箱等，这些设备的干燥效果和干燥能力较自然干燥明显提高。目前还有用太阳能干燥技术的，此种设备不仅能保证饮片质量，而且可节约大量的能源，降低生产成本。

6. Research on processing equipment

For a long time, PCHM mainly relies on manual operation, with small production scale and large individual differences, and the quality of decoction pieces is difficult to control. Therefore, to achieve the standardization and scale of production of decoction pieces, the research on processing equipment is also an important content of processing research.

Some mechanical equipment was applied or developed gradually after the 1960s.

For the cleaning system, manual operation is replaced by a variety of electric machiner in recent years. For the washing equipment, at present, there are several kinds of washing machines, such as drum type, scraper type, and chain plate type. For the softening processing, there is a decompression cold-soaking softening device, which can not only make the medicinal materials meet the softening requirements, but also ensure the quality of the pieces, and improve the working efficiency about 30 times. It can shorten the softening time of medicinal materials and ensure the quality of decoction pieces by using a multi-function extraction tank. For the cutting equipment, there are mainly chopping knives and a rotary cutting machine.

For the frying equipment, a simple sprinkler device is added to the drum-type frying machine, which can be used for the processing of medicinal materials with liquid assistant materials. The modification of three different speed governor for the rotary drum type frying machine can meet the temperature requirements of all kinds of traditional Chinese medicine processing, such as different types of frying machine, infrared frying machine, electric heating type frying machine, electronic control frying machine, and computer frying machine, etc. The electronic program-controlled frying machine adopts the sequence controller, which enables the automatic operation of feeding, frying, discharging, sifting, wind selecting, blowing cold, and packing The computer frying medicine machine adopts the electronic computer terminal control system, has the baking heating, the constant temperature, the programmed heating function, by the computer input each fried medicine craft parameter, realizes the automatic open door feed, the automatic control stirring speed and the opening and stopping automatically to spray quantitative liquid assistant material, the automatically exhausting smoke, automatically opening door to discharge. It is also equipped with a process recording instrument, the process data can be stored and recorded, the process data and working conditions can also be displayed in the terminal screen with Chinese, and operating with Chinese question and answer type. In the event of mechanical failure, there are electrical protection and alarm devices, equipped with two sets of automatic and manual process control systems. The machine is suitable for various processing.

For the drying of decoction pieces, commonly used are flip plate dryer, hot air dryer, far-infrared radiation drying box, and so on, the drying effect and drying ability of this equipment are improved compared with natural drying. There is also solar drying technology, such equipment can not only guarantee the quality of pieces but also save a lot of energy, reduce production costs.

7. 中药相关产品的研究

（1）中药配方颗粒的研究：中药配方颗粒是指单味中药饮片经水提取浓缩而制成的颗粒。其目的不是替代中药饮片，而是适应市场需求而对饮片的补充。因其不能单独使用，只供中医临床配制处方用，所以在名称前加"配方"二字，以示与一般中成药颗粒剂相区别。

中药配方颗粒作为中药饮片相关产品，具有不少优点（如不须临用时煎煮等），为急诊提供了方便快捷的中药；随服随冲，使用简单；促进了饮片行业及中药材生产的规范化、标准化；利于配方电脑调控自动化；还能适应国际市场对植物药提取物的需要，其附加值比出口药材高得多。但是，中医处方以中药配方颗粒配制，不一定与传统饮片制得的汤剂等效。传统饮片制备汤剂，有先煎、后下等特殊处理，方药合煎是一个极复杂的过程，可能会发生酸碱中和、取代、水解、聚合、缩合、氧化、变性等化学反应。方药单煎后合并使用，不完全等效于方药的群煎使用，这也是汤剂剂型改进的难点所在。

中药配方颗粒实质上就是"单味药浸膏颗粒"，它应该是不仅可供配方用，也可单独使用。如果一定要限定为"中药配方颗粒"，那就起码应做颗粒与原饮片相应剂量主要药效学和（或）毒性的对比实验。中药配方颗粒应有规范的质量标准，其内容应包括：药品名称、来源、炮制、制法、性状、鉴别、检查、浸出物、含量测定、功能与主治、用法与用量、注意、规格、贮藏、有效期等项目。

（2）中药超微粉的研究：中药超微粉系指采用超微粉体技术将中药饮片粉碎成一定粒径的粉体。超微粉继承了中药"散剂""煮散""袋泡剂"的优点，保留了中药或复方的全部组分及其药效学物质基础。粉体可用于加工成颗粒剂、咀嚼片、微囊等中药剂型；或利用其渗透率强等性质，制成外用或透皮制剂；或与超微磁粉制成靶向制剂。

7. Research on TCM related products

(1) Study on TCM formula granules: TCM formulation granules refers to the granules through water extraction and concentration of a single decoction piece of TCM. Its purpose is not to replace the traditional Chinese medicine pieces, but to adapt to the market demand for the supplement of the pieces. Because it cannot be used alone, only for TCM clinical preparation of prescription, so before the name adding "formula" to show the difference with the general Chinese patent medicine granules.

As a related product of TCM, TCM Formula Granules have many advantages (such as not needing decoction at the time of clinical use, etc.), which provide provides convenience and quick for clinical emergency use, easy use either. It promotes the normalization and standardization of the decoction pieces industry and production of traditional Chinese medicine, facilitates the automation of formulation through computer regulation, and can also meet the needs of the international market for plant medicine extracts, and its added value is much higher than that of exported medicinal materials. However, the TCM prescription prepared with formulation granules is not necessarily equivalent to the traditionally prepared decoction. Traditional decoction prepared is sometimes with special treatments such as first decoction and then lower decoction. It is a very complex process, acid and alkali neutralization, substitution, hydrolysis, polymerization, condensation, oxidation, denaturation, and other chemical reactions may occur during decocting. The combination of decoctions of a single piece is not entirely equivalent to the group decoction of prescription, which is also the difficulty of improving the form of decoction.

TCM formulation granule is essentially "single medicine extract granule ", it should be not only available for the formulation but also can be used alone. If it must be limited to "TCM formula granules ", then at least should do the corresponding dose of granules and the original decoction of the main pharmacodynamics and/or toxicity of the comparative test. The quality standards of TCM should include, drug name, source, processing method, character, identification, inspection, extract, content determination, function and main treatment, usage, and dosage, attention, specification, storage, validity period, etc.

(2) Research on the ultrafine powder of TCM: The ultrafine powder of TCM refers to the use of ultrafine powder technology to crush Chinese medicine pieces into a certain size of the powder. Ultrafine powder inherits the advantages of TCM "powder" and "boil powder" and "drug bag", and retains the whole component of TCM or compound and its pharmacodynamic material basis. The powder can be used for processing into granules, chewable tablets, microcapsules, and other TCM dosage forms, or make use of its strong penetration rate and other properties, made into external use or transdermal preparations, or to make the preparation with ultrafine magnetic powder.

超微粉的细胞破壁率高，加快了活性成分的溶出、提高溶出率，使吸收速度和程度增大从而提高中药制剂的效应强度和起效速度。药物的比表面积增大，吸收速度和程度提高，可减少用药剂量，节约原料药材，尤其适用于濒危中药材，有利于中医药的持续发展。但是超微粉还存在不少需要研究的问题，例如，中药属性（矿物类、植物类、动物类）、入药部位、活性成分性质、药材含湿量等不同，如何选择超微粉碎设备；中药经超微粉碎后，其生物利用度会发生改变，必然导致其疗效与毒性改变，是否还按照《中国药典》规定的剂量使用，应研究确定；超微粉体给中药的应用带来了优势，但也给后续制剂工艺带来了困难，例如，提取时易糊化、滤过困难，制备固体制剂时，易结聚、黏附、吸湿，制粒、成型困难，因此对超微粉体进行表面改性的研究成为热点；超微粉碎产业化推广的主要阻力是生产成本高，仅适用于高附加值产品的应用。此外，超微粉的粒径小，表面积大，表面活性强，其可燃性、氧化性、静电结聚性也增强，尤其是干法粉碎使超微粉的粒度在 10μm 以下时，极易燃烧、爆炸。因此，如何从粉碎设备设计、粉碎工艺选择、物料处理、环境等方面消除产生静电、火花、积热等隐患，以及提高超微粉碎的安全性，都是值得关注的课题。

综上所述，目前中药炮制研究在许多方面已取得了较好的成果。传统的炮制经验基本得到了传承与发展；炮制历史文献资料得到了整理，这为中药炮制研究的选题、设计奠定了基础；部分中药炮制的作用原理得到了初步阐明，为改进炮制工艺、制订饮片质量标准提供了依据；炮制设备也由半机械化向机械化、自动化、信息化逐步过渡；中药配方颗粒、超微粉等是中药药剂有关理论、方法、技术设备在中药炮制中的应用，在一定程度上促进了中药饮片工业的发展。

The cell wall-breaking rate of ultrafine powder is high, which accelerates the dissolution of active components, improves the dissolution rate, and increases the absorption rate and degree, thus increasing the effect strength and onset rate of TCM preparations. The specific surface area of drugs increases, the absorption speed and degree increase, which can reduce the dosage of drugs, save raw materials and medicinal materials, especially suitable for endangered Chinese medicinal materials, which is conducive to the sustainable development of TCM. However, there are still many problems that need to be studied in ultrafine powder, for example, how to choose the ultrafine crushing equipment with different properties of TCM (minerals, plants, animals), the parts of medicines, the properties of active ingredients, the moisture content of medicinal materials, etc. After ultrafine crushing, the bioavailability of drugs will change, which will inevitably lead to changes in curative effect and toxicity. Whether it is also used by the dosage specified in the *Chinese Pharmacopoeia* should be studied and determined. The ultrafine powder brings advantages to the application of TCM, but it also brings difficulties to the subsequent preparation process. For example, it is easy to gelatinize and filter when extracting, and it is easy to gather, adhere, absorb moisture, granulate, and form when preparing solid preparation, so the research on surface modification of ultrafine powder has become a hot topic. The main resistance to the promotion of ultrafine crushing industrialization is the high production cost, which is only suitable for the application of high value-added products, in addition, the particle size of the ultrafine powder is small, the specific surface area is large, the surface activity is strong, and its flammability, oxidation and electrostatic agglomeration are also enhanced, especially when the particle size of the ultrafine powder is below 10um by dry grinding, it is easy to burn and explode. Therefore, how to eliminate the hidden dangers of static electricity, sparks, heat accumulation, and so on from the aspects of crushing equipment design, crushing process selection, material treatment, environment, and so on, and to improve the safety of ultrafine crushing are all the subjects of concern.

To sum up, Chinese medicine processing research has achieved good results in many aspects. The traditional processing experience has been inherited and developed; the historical documents have been sorted out, which has laid a foundation for the selection and design of traditional Chinese medicine processing research; the principle of some traditional Chinese medicine processing has been preliminarily clarified, which has provided the basis for improving the processing technology and formulating the quality standard of decoction pieces; the processing equipment has also been gradually transitioned from semi-mechanization to mechanization, automation, and informationization; the TCM formula granules and ultra-fine powder are the application of traditional Chinese medicine pharmaceutical theory, method and technical equipment in the processing of TCM, which has promoted the application of traditional Chinese medicine decoction pieces of the industry to a certain extent development.

三、中药炮制研究的方法

1. 选题原则

选择科研课题，即确定科研的主攻方向和具体目标，是科研的起点和关键。选题的程序及原则与其他领域的研究选题基本相同，必须坚持实用性、可行性、科学性、创新性、效益性的选题原则。

（1）**实用性**：就科学技术是第一生产力而言，科研选题不能离开社会的需要，否则难以权衡其价值。对中药炮制研究的选题来说，首先应选择毒性药材进行研究，其次选择贵重药材、传统认为炮制前后作用差异较大的药材、炭药，以及药材已知成分和药理作用与中医所说的药效接近的品种。只有了解了这些药物炮制前后理化性质和药理作用的变化，以及这些变化的临床意义，才能正确地指导和促进炮制方法的改进，制订饮片质量标准，提高药品质量，确保临床用药有效安全。

（2）**可行性**：坚持选题的可行性或可能性原则，即考虑完成课题的条件。选题时分析课题的难易程度，预期达到课题目标所必须具备的客观条件，要从研究方案、课题组织、研究人员组成、仪器设备、研究经费、主客观条件的相互结合与联系等方面进行综合考虑。对中药炮制研究来说，科研人员必须有较坚实的中医药学基础，同时具有一定的现代科学知识和技能。只有将中医药传统理论、经验与现代科学知识、技能结合起来，其研究成果才有价值。

Section Three The Methods of PCHM Research

1. The principles of choosing topics

Choosing scientific research topics, that is, determining the main direction and specific objectives of scientific research is the starting point and key to scientific research. The procedure and principle of selecting topics are the same as that of other research, the principles of practicability, feasibility, science, innovation, and benefit must be persisted.

(1) The principle of practicality: As far as science and technology is the first productive force, scientific research topics cannot leave the needs of society, otherwise, it is difficult to weigh their value. For the selected topics of PCHM research, the research on toxic medicinal materials processing should be first chosen, and then the precious medicinal materials, the traditional medicinal materials which are considered changed a lot before and after processing, the charcoal drugs, and the pieces whose ingredients and pharmacological effects are close to the pharmacological effect of traditional Chinese medicines. Only by understanding the changes of physicochemical properties and pharmacological effects before and after processing, and the clinical significance of these changes, can we correctly guide and promote the improvement of the processing methods, formulate the quality standards of decoction pieces, improve the quality of medicine, and ensure the clinical safety and efficacy of these drugs.

(2) The principle of feasibility: Adhere to the principle of feasibility or possibility of the topic, that is, consider the conditions for the completion of the topic. When selecting the topic, we should analyze the difficulty of the subject, and expect the objective conditions to be met, and consider the research plan, the organization of the topic, the composition of the researcher, the instruments and equipment, the research funds, and the combination and connection of the subjective and objective conditions. For the research of PCHM, researchers must have a solid knowledge of TCM, and at the same time have certain modern scientific knowledge and skills. Only by combining TCM theory, experience with modern scientific knowledge and skills can the research results be valuable.

（3）科学性：科学研究必须具有科学性，科学性的核心是实事求是，违背事实和客观规律就没有科学研究的意义。目前中药炮制研究选题多数是验证传统炮制理论和方法，这是正确的，但其中也有的是误传误用。例如，《中国药典》1985年版规定龟以腹甲入药，名为龟板。经对部分历史文献资料调查，元代、明代以前，龟上甲与下甲皆可入药，后因种种原因龟上甲被废弃。因此，从龟上、下甲能否等重量替代入药，入汤剂时以何种方法炮制饮片等问题开展系统研究，其成果为恢复龟上甲药用提供了文献依据和实验依据。《中国药典》从1990年版起规定龟以背甲（上甲）及腹甲（下甲）入药，名为龟甲。由此看来，选题必须进行广泛深入的调查和课题检索，在反复分析研究的基础上，慎重地确定科研课题。

（4）创新性：在科学技术发展成为人类重要活动的今天，经济竞争归根到底是科学技术发展的速度和水平的竞争。因此，课题是否具有竞争性是关键问题。要充分考虑中药炮制研究是否是一种创新性的工作，研究的指标和方法是否符合中医药理论，是否充分利用现代科学知识和手段，有无自己的设计特色。目前，将中药炮制纳入方剂中进行研究的选题思路值得借鉴，因为方剂是调整体内系统平衡的最优化治疗系统，也是中医临床用药的一大特点。

(3) The principle of scientific: Scientific research must be scientific, the core of science is to seek truth from facts, there is no scientific significance if research is contrary to facts and objective laws. At present, most of the research topics are to verify the traditional processing theory and methods, which is correct, but some of them are misused. For example, the 1985 edition of the *Chinese Pharmacopoeia* stipulated that tortoises should be used in medicine as ventral beetles. Before the Yuan Dynasty and Ming Dynasty, the turtle upper and lower armor could be used in medicine, but turtle upper armor was discarded for various reasons. Therefore, whether the same weight of the upper and lower tortoise can be used alternative, what is the best way to prepare the decoction pieces, based on the above questions to do systematic research, the results would provide the literature and experimental basis for the recovery use of turtle upper armor. Since the 1990 edition of the *Chinese Pharmacopoeia*, the *Chinese Pharmacopoeia* has stipulated that tortoises should be used in medicine for their backs (upper armor) and abdomen (lower armor). Therefore, it is necessary to determine the research topic to carry out extensive and in-depth investigation and subject retrieval based on repeated analysis and research.

(4) The principle of innovation: With the development of science and technology becoming an important activity of mankind, economic competition is, in the final analysis, the speed and level of science and technology development. Therefore, whether the subject is competitive or not is the key issue. It is necessary to fully consider whether the research of PCHM is an innovative work, whether the indexes and methods of the research are under the theory of TCM, whether to make full use of modern scientific knowledge and means, and whether they have their design characteristics. At present, it is a worth reference that including the research of PCHM into the research of the prescription, because the prescription is the optimal treatment system to adjust the balance of the body system, and it is also a major feature of the clinical use of TCM.

（5）效益性：效益主要包括科学效益、社会效益和经济效益。所谓科学效益就是选题对学科在学术上、科学价值上的推动作用。科学效益是社会效益和经济效益的基础和保证。对中药炮制研究来说，由于中药炮制受历史条件和科学文化水平的限制，其炮制方法比较原始，工艺比较简单，理论阐述亦较简略，如果不探讨中药炮制的科学内涵和临床意义，就不能指导和促进炮制方法的改进，也就难以体现科学效益。例如，药材"去芦"问题，历代医药学家认为"芦"为非药用部位，有的且"能吐人"，故应去除。通常认为要去芦的药材有数十种，其中就包括人参。因为人参贵重，参芦占全人参药材的12%～15%，弃之可惜。为此，有研究对人参芦与人参主根进行系统比较，结果产生了较好的科学效益，而且对参芦的综合开发利用会带来很大的社会效益和经济效益。经化学成分、药理和毒理研究，以及临床观察，结果皆表明，人参芦与人参主根中人参皂苷的种类基本相同，但含量却比主根高2～3倍，挥发油亦比主根高3倍多。参芦具有与主根和全参相同的药理作用，对实验动物有相似的抗疲劳、耐缺氧、耐高温、耐低温、抗利尿、镇痛等作用。参芦与人参根、参芦总皂苷与人参根总皂苷具有相似的降低心率和血管阻力、增加血流量、提高实验动物各种组织中Na^+-K^+-ATP酶活性、抑制Mg^{2+}-ATP酶活性的作用；对cAMP和cGMP的含量具有双向调节作用。目前尚未发现参芦的化学成分中含有催吐成分，对催吐药物敏感的动物，如猫、狗、猴等，均没有表现出对人参芦的敏感性。参芦与主根的急性和亚急性毒性实验结果也相似，故《中国药典》1995年版已改为人参不去芦。

2. 选题途径

（1）从当前炮制研究存在的问题选题：中药炮制研究选题，首先应对当前选题的动态趋势及存在的问题等进行认真的调查研究，才能广开思路，找准目标。从公开报道的资料中就可以发现炮制研究存在的问题，有如下几个方面。

(5) The principle of benefits: Benefits mainly include scientific, social, and economic benefits. The so-called scientific benefit is the promotion of the topic to the academic and scientific value of the subject. The scientific benefit is the basis and guarantee of social benefit and economic benefit. For the research of PCHM, it is limited by the historical conditions and scientific and cultural level, its processing method is relatively primitive, the technology is relatively simple, and the theory is also relatively brief. If we do not explore the scientific connotation and clinical significance of PCHM, we cannot guide and promote the improvement of processing methods, and it is difficult to reflect the scientific benefits. For example, the problem of "discarding the reed head" of medicinal materials, the past pharmacists thought that "reed head" was a non-medicinal part, some of them "making people vomit", so should be removed. There are dozens of herbs commonly thought to discarding the reed head, including ginseng. Because ginseng is valuable, there are 12% to 15% reed heads of the whole ginseng medicinal materials, if the reed head is abandoned it's a pity. Therefore, the main roots of ginseng and ginseng reed head have been systematically compared, the results not only produce good, the development and utilization of ginseng and ginseng reed head also bring great social and economic benefits. Through chemical composition, pharmacology, and toxicology studies, as well as clinical observation, the results showed that the species of ginsenoside in the main root of ginseng and ginseng reed head were the same, but the content was 2~3 times higher than that of the main root, and the volatile oil was more than 3 times higher than that of the main root. The ginseng reed head has the same pharmacological action as the main root and the whole ginseng and has similar anti-fatigue, anti-anoxia, high-temperature resistance, low-temperature resistance, anti-diuretic, and analgesic effects on the experimental animals. The ginseng reed head and main root, the total saponins of ginseng reed head, and ginseng root have the similar effect of decreasing heart rate and vascular resistance, increasing blood flow, increasing Na^+-K^+-ATPase activity, and inhibiting Mg^{2+}-ATPase activity. There is a bidirectional regulatory effect on the content of cAMP and cGMP. It has not been found that the chemical constituents of the ginseng reed head contain vomiting ingredients, and the animals that are sensitive to vomit drugs, cats, dogs, monkeys, and ginseng reed head, all showed no vomiting effect. The results of the acute and subacute toxicity tests were similar. Therefore, the *Chinese Pharmacopoeia* 1995 edition has been changed to not discard ginseng reed head.

2. Ways to choose topics

(1) Selecting topics on problems in current processing research: First of all, to select the PCHM research topics, it is necessary to investigate the current topic of the dynamic trends, as well as the existing problems, which will open up our ideas and help us to find the right goal. From the publicly reported information can find research problems in the PCHM, such as following several aspects.

①**对同一种中药的炮制研究结论截然不同**：例如，有研究认为乳香所含树脂是活血镇痛的主要成分，应炮制去油药用；也有研究认为其镇痛作用的有效成分是挥发油，应生用或提取挥发油药用。

②**对同一种中药选用何种辅料炮制，看法不一**：例如，延胡索《中国药典》2020年版仍收载醋炙或醋煮延胡索，因为醋炙延胡索水煎液中总生物碱量较酒炙品高出一倍多。但又有报道醋炙、酒炙延胡索均能提高其水煎液中生物碱和延胡索乙素的煎出量，其止痛作用酒炙仅次于醋炙和酒蒸。酒蒸能否代替醋炙，值得进一步研究。

③**对同一种中药选用何种炮制工艺，看法不一**：例如，对白芍的加工，《中国药典》2015年版规定芍药采后洗净，除去头尾及细根，置沸水中煮后除去外皮或去皮后再煮，晒干。但据报道，未经加工的原芍药含芍药苷为3.02%，而去皮后降为1.49%，认为白芍不必刮皮。亦有报道认为，芍药外皮中不仅含有与白芍相同的化学成分，也含有其不具有的化学成分，因此，白芍是否要去外皮尚须深入研究。

④**对炮制程度缺乏客观指标**：目前多数中药炮制程度仍靠传统经验，缺乏客观指标。如对熟地黄的炮制方法有单蒸、加酒蒸，酒蒸又有笼蒸、罐炖、九蒸九晒。但炮制程度至黑润，在实际生产中很难掌握一致。有报道，地黄中梓醇的存在是其晒干或蒸干变黑的原因，并且梓醇具有降血糖、利尿、缓泻作用。因此，目前至少可根据经验，再结合梓醇的含量，作为熟地黄炮制质量控制的指标之一。

Part III Modern Research of PCHM

① **The research on the processing of the same traditional Chinese medicine is quite different.** For example, some people think that the resin of Olibanum (Ruxiang) is the main component of activating blood circulation and relieving pain, so the oil in this drug should be removed. Some people think that the effective part with analgesic effect is a volatile oil. The drugs should be used without processing to keep oil or the oil should be extracted for clinical use.

② **Different views on the choice of the processing assistant materials of the same traditional Chinese medicine.** For example, in the 2015 edition of the Chinese Pharmacopoeia, there contains vinegar-fried or vinegar-boiled Corydalis Rhizoma (Yanhusuo), because the total amount of alkaloid in the decoction of vinegar-fried Corydalis Rhizoma is more than double that of the decoction of wine-fried Corydalis Rhizoma. However, it has been reported that vinegar and alcohol processing can all increase the amount of alkaloid and tetrahydropalmatine in the decoction, and the analgesic effect of wine processed Corydalis Rhizoma is second only to vinegar-fried and wine steamed products, Whether wine steaming can replace vinegar frying is worth further study.

③ **Different views on the chosen processing technology of the same traditional Chinese medicine.** For example, for the processing of Paeoniae Radix Alba (Baishao), the 2015 edition of the *Chinese Pharmacopoeia* stipulates that Paeoniae Radix Alba should be washed after harvest, and the head and tail and fine roots should be removed, boiled in boiling water after removing the skin or peeling before processing and then dried. However, it is reported that the peoniflorin in raw Paeoniae Radix Alba is 3.02% compared to 1.49% after peeling, so it is considered that it does not need to peel Paeoniae Radix Alba. It has also been reported that peel of Paeoniae Radix Alba not only contains the same chemical constituents as Paeoniae Radix Alba but also the chemical constituents it does not exist in Paeoniae Radix Alba. Therefore, it needs further study whether the peel of Paeoniae Radix Alba should be discarded.

④ **Lack of objective indicators of the degree of processing.** At present, most of the processing degrees of traditional Chinese medicine still rely on traditional experience, lack objective indicators. Such as prepared Rhizome of adhesive Rehmannia (Shudihuang), the processing methods include steaming, steaming with the wine which includes steaming in cage or pot, repeated steaming and drying several times, But the degree of processing to black is difficult to master in real production. It has been reported that the presence of Catalpol is the cause of drying or drying and blackening of prepared Rhizome of adhesive Rehmannia, and it has the effect of reducing blood sugar, diuretic, and diarrhea. Therefore, the experienced judge combining with the content of Catalpol can be as a quality control index of prepared Rhizome of adhesive Rehmannia.

⑤ **实验研究结果与传统炮制理论不符**：传统炮制理论有精华，也有糟粕，须用现代实验方法验证和发展。如传统认为"泽泻滋阴利水盐水炒"（《得配本草》），但有实验表明，泽泻的生品、酒炙品、麸炒品均有利尿作用，唯独盐制品利尿作用并不明显。可是《中国药典》历次版本皆收载泽泻盐制品。而有研究表明，盐泽泻的利尿作用与酒制泽泻、麸炒泽泻相比并没有明显差异。综上所述，对泽泻盐炙的问题尚须进一步研究。

⑥ **只注意宏量成分，不注意微量成分**：如有实验认为，紫硇砂经醋制后成为较纯的氯化钠，含量达98%以上，因此想利用食盐代替紫硇砂药用。古人认为，硇砂能"消五金八石，腐坏人肠胃"，炮制是"杀其毒及去其尘秽"。现代研究认为，紫硇砂有治疗癌症的作用，其生品对小鼠S180肉瘤有抑制作用，普通食盐是没有此种作用的。因此，认为紫硇砂中抗癌活性成分可能是除NaCl以外的微量离子。这一问题有待进一步研究探讨。

⑦ **不加分析地依法炮制未必完全合理**：目前所说的依法炮制基本上是"遵古炮制"，没有通过现代科学的验证。例如，《中国药典》历次版本皆规定附子采后加工成盐附子、黑顺片、白附片。盐附子入药尚须制成淡附片。据报道，附子采后经水洗、胆巴泡、煮、剥皮、切片、蒸片、烘片等加工炮制处理过程，总生物碱量损失81.30%。附子炮制的目的是减毒，而其毒性与乌头碱的含量不成平行关系，主要决定于双型乌头碱的水解或分解程度。故是否可改用加压蒸法炮制，使双酯型乌头碱类分解成毒性低的苯甲酰单酯型乌头碱类和几乎无毒性的乌头原碱而减毒，值得研究。

⑤ **The experimental results do not conform to the traditional processing theory.** The traditional processing theory has the essence but also has the dross, needs to use the modern experimental method to verify and develop. Such as the traditional thought that "Oriental water plantain rhizome (Zexie) should be stir-frying with saltwater to promote the effect of nourishing yin to promote diuresis "(*Depei Bencao*), but some experiments show that the raw products of Oriental water plantain rhizome, the stir-frying with wine products and stir-frying with bran products all have a diuretic effect, but the diuretic effect of salt water-processed products is not obvious. However, the *Chinese Pharmacopoeia* records the salt water-processed products in every edition. Studies have shown that the diuretic effect of salt water-processed products is not significantly different from that of wine processed and bran processed products. To sum up, the problem of salt water-processed products of Oriental water plantain rhizome needs further study.

⑥ **Pay attention only to macro components, not to trace components.** It is considered that after processing with vinegar, Halite violaceous (Zinaosha) becomes purer sodium chloride with content over 98%. Therefore, salt is thought to be used instead of Halite violaceous. The ancients believed that the Halite violaceous can "eliminate the metal and mineral, damage stomach and make it rot", the purpose of processing is to "remove its poison and filth." Modern research suggests that Halite violaceous has a therapeutic effect on cancer, and its raw product has an inhibitory effect on S180 sarcoma in mice, and common salt has no such effect. Therefore, it is suggested that the anticancer active component in Halite violaceous sand may be trace ions other than NaCl. This issue needs further study.

⑦ **Processing without any analysis may not be entirely reasonable.** At present, the processing according to laws means "according to the ancient processing methods", many of which have not been verified by modern science. For example, Each edition of *Chinese Pharmacopoeia* all stipulates that Aconiti Lateralis Radix Praeparata (Fuzi) are processed into salt, black and white products after harvest. The salt product needs to be made into a bland product. It was reported that the total alkaloid loss of Aconiti Kusnezoffii Radix Lateralis Preparata was 81.30% after washing, gall bladder soaking, boiling, peeling, slicing, steaming, baking, and so on. The purpose of processing is to reduce the toxicity, but its toxicity is not parallel to the content of aconitine, mainly depends on the degree of hydrolysis or decomposition of the double-type aconitine. Therefore, it is worth studying whether to change the processing method to steaming with pressure, making the double-type aconitine being hydrolyzed and decomposed into benzoyl monoester-type aconitine with low toxicity or aconine almost without toxicity.

（2）从中药已知的特种成分入手选题：凡是中药中特种成分性质比较清楚者，就可以寻找到其定性定量方法，进一步对该中药炮制前后此种成分进行分析比较。例如，栀子中除含栀子苷类成分外，尚含熊果酸。熊果酸具有明显的降温与安定作用，为栀子解热除烦的有效成分。可用高效液相色谱法测定栀子不同炮制品中栀子苷和熊果酸的含量。

（3）从中药药效或毒副作用入手选题：中药炮制的目的主要是增强药效或消减其毒副作用。用什么指标来衡量中药药效或毒副作用才符合中医药理论，这是值得探讨的问题。例如，自《神农本草经》以来，黄芪就被认为对痈疽有效，用于排脓。有研究证明，黄芪的抑菌作用强，可以抑菌作用为指标验证黄芪托毒排脓、生肌的科学性。此外，毒性中药一般可分为两种类型，一类是其毒性成分，与治疗成分不一样，须通过炮制将毒性成分去除，如巴豆中巴豆毒素等。另一类既是有毒成分又是治疗成分，要通过炮制使其达到一定的含量，或转变成毒性较低的物质，如马钱子中的马钱子碱和士的宁等。对毒性成分和有效成分尚不清楚的中药，可选择主要药效学和毒理学指标做各种炮制品的对比研究。

（4）从中药配伍理论和技术展开研究：中药配伍应用是中医用药的特点之一，通过配伍可起到增效或解毒等作用。运用中药配伍理论和经验，可以创造出新的炮制品。例如《全国中药炮制规范》1988年版收三黄汤制炉甘石，既是传统炮制品，也为创制新的炮制品提供了思路。有人在研究由黄连、黄柏、大黄、甘草组成的复方对金黄色葡萄球菌代谢的影响过程中发现，黄柏对细菌 RNA 的合成有强烈的抑制作用，大黄对细菌乳酸脱氢酶的抑制最强，黄连强烈抑制细菌呼吸和核酸的合成。推想以三黄汤制炉甘石是从多种途径影响细菌的代谢环节、可增强炉甘石生肌消炎的作用。

(2) Starting with the known special components of traditional Chinese medicine: Where the nature of special components in traditional Chinese medicine is relatively clear, we can find a qualitative and quantitative method to analyze and compare these components before and after processing. For example, the Gardeniae Fructus (Zhizi) contains geniposideursolic and ursolic acid which has the obvious effects of stability and cooling. And the ursolic acid is the affective component of anti-heat, cooling in Fructus Gardeniae fruit. The content of geniposideursolic and ursolic acid in different processed products can be determined by HPLC.

(3) Choose the topic from the medicine effect or side effect of traditional Chinese medicine: The main purpose of PCHM is to enhance herbal medicines' efficacy or reduce their side effects. It is worth discussing what index is used to measure the efficacy or side effects of TCM to conform to the traditional theories. For example, since the *Shennong Herbal Classic*, Astragali Radix (Huangqi) has been considered to be effective for the discharge of pus. Some studies have proved that Astragali Radix has a strong bacteriostasis effect, which can be used as an index to verify the scientific nature of the discharge of pus and muscle. In addition, some Chinese medicine with toxicity can generally be divided into two types, one is their toxic components, not the same as the treatment components, must be processed to remove toxic components, such as croton toxin in Fructus Crotonis, and so on. The other is the component is both toxic and therapeutic, which should be processed to remove to a certain level, or turned into less toxic components, such as strychnine in Strychni Semen. For the herbal medicines whose toxic components and active components are unknown, the main pharmacodynamic and toxicological indicators can be selected for the comparative study of various processed products.

(4) Starting the research on the theory and technology of TCM: The application of compatibility of medicines is one of the characteristics of TCM, through compatibility the medicines can synergistic or detoxification. With the compatibility theory and experience, new processed products can be created. For example, the Calamina (Luganshi) processed with sanhuang decoction recorded in the 1988 edition of the *National Standard for the Processing of Traditional Chinese Herbal Medicine* is not only the traditional processed product but also provides ideas for creating new kinds of processed products. In the course of studying the effect of the compound composed of Goptidis Rhizoma (Huanglian), Phellodendri Chinensis Cortex (Huangbai), Rhei Radix Et Rhizoma (Daihuang), and Glycyrrhizae Radix Et Rhizoma (Gancao) on the metabolism of Staphylococcus aureus, it was found that Phellodendri Chinensis Cortex had a strong inhibitory effect on the synthesis of bacterial RNA, and Rhei Radix Et Rhizoma had the strongest inhibition on the dehydrolactic acid of bacteria, and Coptidis Rhizoma strongly inhibited the respiration of bacteria and the synthesis of nucleic acid. It is assumed that the Calamina processed with sanhuang decoction can enhance the effect of anti-inflammatory and promoting granulation through influencing the metabolism of bacteria in many ways.

（5）**从历代医药典籍中寻找课题**：阅读历代医药典籍不仅是搜集炮制历史沿革资料所必需，而且也是进行炮制研究选题的一种重要途径。例如，自古以来认为半夏生品有毒，能"戟人咽""令人吐"，须以水长期浸漂去毒。清代赵学敏在《本草纲目拾遗》中曾指出："今药肆所售仙半夏，惟将半夏浸泡，尽去其汁味……全失本性……是无异食半夏渣滓，何益之有？"从实验亦可看出，半夏有毒物质不溶或难溶于水，短期浸泡不能达到去毒的目的，长期浸泡则水溶性成分损失达88.1%，醇溶成分损失87.5%、生物碱损失50%。有报道认为半夏经高温或高压处理，均能破坏其毒性且工艺简便。在半夏有效成分和有毒成分尚存争议的情况下，半夏的水浸泡工艺能否用高温高压替代，值得深入研究。

（6）**将其他学科理论和技术引进炮制学**：可应用化学、药理学、微生物学、免疫学、生物化学、物理学等近代科学技术，对中药炮制原理、方法、工艺等方面进行研究。例如，采用薄层层析和UV-3000紫外分光光度法，以及高效液相色谱仪等测定白芍5种炮制品中芍药苷、丹皮酚、苯甲酸的含量；用化学动力学方法建立何首乌清蒸过程中成分随时间变化的动力学方程；用免疫学方法探讨大黄对人血清抗原抗体反应及抗体形成作用的影响；用酶学理论和技术对大黄4种不同炮制品中胰蛋白酶、胃蛋白酶、胰脂肪酶、胰淀粉酶的活性进行测定等，皆取得了可喜的成果。

(5) Searching for subjects from past medical books: Reading the classics of the past medical books is not only necessary to collect information about the history of PCHM, but also an important way to make research topics. For example, since ancient times it is believed that Corydalis Rhizoma (Banxia) is toxic, which can "irritate throat", "emetic effect", need to be long-term water bleaching to remove poison. In the Qing Dynasty, Zhao Xuemin pointed out in the *Supplement of Compendium of Materia Medica* (*Bencao Gangmu Shiyi*), " This medicine shop sells Corydalis Rhizoma, but soaks the Corydalis Rhizoma until its taste lost, which makes the effect reduce and have no benefit", It can also be seen from the experiment that the toxic substance of Corydalis Rhizoma is insoluble or soluble in water very difficult, and the short-term soaking cannot achieve the purpose of detoxification. The loss of water-soluble components in long-term soaking is 88.1%, the loss of alcohol-soluble components is 87.5%, and the loss of alkaloid is 50%. It has been reported that the toxicity of Corydalis Rhizoma can be destroyed by high temperature or high-pressure treatment, and the process is simple. Whether the water soaking process of Corydalis Rhizoma can be replaced by high temperature and high-pressure processing is worthy of further study.

(6) Introducing theories and techniques of other disciplines into processing: Modern science and technology, such as chemistry, pharmacology, microbiology, immunology, biochemistry, and physics, can be used to study the processing mechanism, methods, and techniques of PCHM. For example, the content of paeoniflorin, paeonol, and benzoic acid in Paeoniae Radix Alba (Baishao) were determined by TLC, UV-3000 UV spectrophotometry, and high-performance liquid chromatography. The kinetic equation of the composition of Polygonum Multiflorum Radix (Heshouwu) was established by the chemical kinetic method. The effect of Rhei Radix Et Rhizoma on the anti-antibody reaction and antibody formation in human serum was investigated by the immunological method. The activity of trypsin, protease, trypsin, amylase, and amylase in four different products of Rhei Radix Et Rhizoma (Daihuang) was determined by enzyme theory and technique. All of these have achieved gratifying results.

3. 实验设计

（1）设计方法

①以中医临床疗效为设计的出发点：中药的作用是中医药工作者在长期的临床实践中积累总结出来的。对中药作用的认识和研究，绝不能拘泥于某种单纯的化学成分或纯化学成分的某种药理模型进行研究，而忽视中药的特性。例如，中药四季青内服有清热解毒的作用，但体外实验却无抑菌作用。因此，用什么指标来衡量中药药效或毒副作用才能符合中医药理论，这是值得探讨的问题。又如清热解毒类中药的抗感染作用往往不是因为它们有直接的抗微生物作用，而是与其免疫调节有关。再如，麦芽、神曲、山楂、鸡内金等消导药，习惯上皆炒至焦香后入药，如果以所含酵素类成分来解释它们的消食作用，就具有很大的局限性。因为淀粉酶、蛋白酶等经加热炒制后或入煎剂会遭到破坏，即使不被完全破坏，经口服后在胃酸的作用下，淀粉酶（最适合的 pH 为 6.8）也会失活。有的药物炒至焦香后，亦具有一定的苦味，轻微的苦味能对舌尖味觉神经及胃肠黏膜产生一种缓和的刺激作用，通过反射机能可纠正部分胃肠衰弱现象，以改善消化功能。如果单用化学成分或药理指标来研究和评价中药炮制的作用则不够完善，必须以中医临床疗效为依据，设计适宜的成分指标和药理实验模型。

②以"证"的模型研究中药炮制原理：辨证论治是中医的特点，而证是根据患者整体宏观表现归纳总结出来的。同病可以异证，因而须异治；异病也可以同证，因而须同治。目前，中药炮制药理研究中，多数以"症"为基础。因此，有些研究结果不能令人信服。如镇痛实验常用"小鼠热板法"或"小鼠醋酸扭体法"，对延胡索的活血止痛、木香的理气止痛、肉桂的散寒止痛、独活的祛风止痛等是否皆适合，答案可能是否定的。再如，大多数炭药用于止血，因此，人们多以出血、凝血时间为指标来研究炭药，但出血原因有很多，有因血热妄行而出血，有因瘀血而出血，有因脾不统血而出血，有因阴虚阳亢而出血，又有外伤性出血、消化道出血、呼吸道出血等，应全面考虑才能充分阐释炭药的炮制机制。

3. Experimental design

(1) Design technique

① Taking the clinical effect of TCM as the starting point of design: The role of TCM is summed up in the long-term clinical practice of TCM workers. The understanding and research of the action of traditional Chinese medicines must not stick to the study of a certain pharmacological model of the chemical component or a pure chemical component, but ignore the characteristics of TCM. For example, traditional Chinese medicine Sijiqing has the effect of clearing away heat and detoxifying through orally taking, but in vitro experiments, it has no bacteriostasis effect. Therefore, what index is used to measure the efficacy or side effects of traditional Chinese medicines to conform to the theory of TCM, which is worth discussing? The anti-infective effect of anti-pyrolysis drugs is not because they have the direct anti-microbial effect, but because of their immune regulation. Another example, malt, koji, hawthorn, chicken gold, and other digestant drugs, all used after stir-frying, if the enzyme-containing components were used to explain their digestion, there has a great limitation. Because after heating and frying or decocting, the amylase, protease, and so on will be destroyed, even if not destroyed, after oral administration, in the action of stomach acid, the amylase (the most suitable pH of 6.8) will be inactivated. Some drugs have a certain bitter taste after fried to coke with fragrance, slight bitter can produce a mild irritation to the tongue's taste nerve and gastrointestinal mucosa, and some gastrointestinal weakness can be corrected by this reflex function, thus improving the digestive function. It is not perfect to study and evaluate the effect of PCHM with chemical composition or pharmacological index alone, it is necessary to design a suitable component index and pharmacological experimental model based on the clinical effects of traditional Chinese medicines.

② Study on the processing principle of TCM with the model of "Syndrome": Treatment based on syndrome differentiation is the characteristics of TCM, and the syndrome is summed up based on the overall macro performance of patients. The same disease can be different syndromes, so must be different treatment; different diseases can also be the same syndrome, so must be the same treatment. At present, most of the pharmacological studies of PCHM are based on "disease". Therefore, some of the findings are not convincing. Such as is it all right to use the common analgesia experiment of "mouse hot plate method" or "mouse acetic acid writhing method", to test the effect of promoting blood circulation to arrest pain of Corydalis Rhizoma (Yanhusuo), the effect of regulating qi to alleviate the pain of Aucklandiae Radix (Muxiang), the effect of eliminating cold to stop the pain of Cinnamon Cortex (Rougui), the effect of dispelling wind to relieve the pain of Angelicae Pubescentis Radix (Duhuo), etc. the answer may be no. Another example, most of the charcoal drugs are used to stop bleeding, so people always take bleeding and blood clotting time as the index to study charcoal medicine, but there are many reasons for bleeding, due to blood fever, blood stasis, spleen disorder, Yin deficiency, and Yang hyperactivity, traumatic bleeding, gastrointestinal bleeding, respiratory bleeding, etc. So comprehensive consideration should be given to fully explain the processing mechanism of carbon medicine.

此外，临床上发现，热证病人的交感神经-肾上腺系统机能活动增强，而寒证病人则相反。经研究表明，用寒凉药（黄连、黄芩、黄柏等）长期喂养大鼠也可出现交感神经-肾上腺系统机能活动降低现象，造成"寒证"模型，而用温热药（附子、干姜、肉桂等）喂养大鼠，则该系统的机能活动增强，造成"热证"模型。这样的动物模型，为研究中药炮制开阔了思路，提供了借鉴。

③**将中药炮制纳入方剂中进行研究**：方剂是调整体内系统平衡的重要手段，也是中医临床用药的一大特点。药物通过配伍组方可起到增效、减毒、缓和药性或产生新药效等作用。单味中药的研究结果往往与该药在方剂中的研究结果不会完全一致，有的甚至截然相反。这也是中药炮制研究成果不易推广应用的原因之一。有报道将白芍的炮制纳入芍药甘草汤中进行研究，发现甘草可提高方中芍药苷的煎出量。白芍生品或清炒品、麸炒品芍药苷含量高，炮制品之间无显著差异，但麸炒白芍的芍甘汤中苯甲酸含量最低，故对脾胃虚弱患者似更适宜。研究提示将炮制纳入方剂种开展整体研究将更有助于临床应用。

（2）设计原则

①**坚持均对照、随机化和重复的原则**：实验设计时应坚持均衡对照，随机化和重复的原则。

对照的设计要按照"齐同对比"的原则，即除了将要探索的因素之外，研究组与对照组的各种条件要尽可能相同，这样才能对比。有人用生药 10g 与该药的炭药 10g 做出血、凝血时间的比较，以说明该药制炭后止血效果是增强还是减弱，这就不是齐同对比。因为生药 10g，制炭后不能得到炭药 10g。目前普遍存在的是对用不同方法或不同辅料炮制的各种炮制品，不按各种炮制品得率和水分折算取样，而是各种炮制品的取样量与原生药等量，这实际上并不是齐同对比。

In addition, from clinically finding, patients with fever syndrome have increased sympathetic-adrenergic system activity, whereas those with the cold syndrome have the opposite. The results showed that the long-term feeding of medicines with cool and cold properties (Goptidis Rhizoma-Huanglian, Scutellariae Radix-Huangqin, Phellodendri Chinensis Cortex-Huangbai, etc.) could also lead to the decrease of the sympathetic function of an adrenal system, resulting in a 'cold syndrome' model. Whereas feeding rats with medicines with warm and hot properties (Aconiti Lateralis Radix Praeparata-Fuzi, Zingiberis Rhizoma-Ganjiang, Cinnamon Cortex-Rougui, etc.), the functional activity of the system was enhanced, resulting in a 'hot syndrome' model. Such animal models provide reference to the study on the PCHM and broaden the thinking.

③ **To study the PCHM in the prescription:** Prescription is an important means to adjust the balance of the body system, but also a major feature of TCM clinical medication. The drugs can be used to increase efficiency, reduce toxicity, moderate the properties of drugs or produce new drugs. The research results of single traditional Chinese herbal medicine are often not completely consistent with the research results of this medicine in the prescription, some even opposed it. This is also one of the reasons why the research results of PCHM are not easy to be popularized and applied. It has been reported that the processing of Paeoniae Radix Alba (Baishao) was studied in paeoniflorin liquorice decoction. It was found that Glycyrrhizae Radix Et Rhizoma can increase the content of paeoniflorin. The content of paeoniae paeoniflorin was high with the raw product, stir-frying product, or stir-frying with bran product in this prescription, and there no significant difference between these processed products, but the content of benzoic acid was the lowest with the stir-frying with bran product in this prescription, so it seemed more suitable for patients with a weak stomach. The research suggests that studying the processed products in the prescription will be more helpful for clinical application.

(2) The points of design

① **Adhere to the principles of control, randomization, and repetition:** The principles of equilibrium control, randomization, and repetition should be adhered to in the design of the test.

The control should be designed under the principle of "uniform contrast", that is, in addition to the factors explored, the study group and the control group should be as much as possible the same conditions, to be able to compare. For example, a comparison of bleeding and clotting time between 10g of raw medicine and 10g of carbon medicine of the drug was made to show whether the hemostatic effect of the drug was enhanced or weakened after charcoal processing. This is not the same contrast, because 10g raw medicine can not get 10g charcoal medicine. At present, it is common to use processed products with different methods or different assistant materials whose sampling amount of various processed products is equal to the amount of primary medicine without counting the yield and moisten of processed products, which is not the same comparison.

随机化就是把研究对象分为几组，使分入研究组与对照组的机会均等，以便使系统误差减少到最低限度。违反随机化原则的做法在炮制研究中常见的有：样品粉碎后只过一种筛目的筛，不规定上下限；取样时不随机化，如动物分组先抓到的（不活泼者）为一组，后抓到的（活泼者）为另一组；实验观察顺序不随机化，等等。做到随机化须要研究者尽最大努力。这是研究者的责任，也反映研究者的科研道德水准。为什么有的研究结果别人不能重复出来，虽然原因很多，但与随机化原则坚持不够有很大关系。

重复是保证科研结果可靠的重要措施之一。重复有两层含义：一是指实验过程是多次重复进行的；二是指设计中提出的方法、结果，别人也能重复出来。有报道认为槐花炒炭后芦丁大量损失，但鞣质增加4倍，并认为槐花炒炭后止血作用增强，可能是鞣质增加的缘故。此后虽然曾有槐花炒炭后鞣质不仅未增加，反而下降的报道，但进一步研究又证明之前的报道是正确的，研究还发现纯芦丁受热后也的确可转化生成鞣质，此种转化与温度和时间密切相关。炮制研究中要得到重现性结果很不容易，与炮制的火候、时间、饮片大小厚薄、样品液的提取条件、实验操作技术等有密切关系。不能根据一两篇实验报道，就轻易否定前人几千年来的炮制理论和技术。

②正确看待和选用数理统计：对科研中所收集到的各种数据要不要使用统计处理，以往存在着两种不同的看法。一种看法认为数理统计万能，把它说得玄而又玄；另一种看法认为数理统计是数学游戏，持怀疑态度，这些都有其片面性。适当地、正确地应用数理统计方法，可以使数据更接近于事实，这对于认识事物的本质是很必要的。

例如有人应用某药治疗手足癣病20例，治愈10例，就得出结论说治愈率为50%。这显然是不可信的，经数理统计处理可知，10/20的实际可能范围是27%~73%（$P=0.05$），而不一定是50%。由此可见，炮制研究中适当地应用数理统计方法是很有必要的，但必须指出，数理统计运用，只能对已得数据进行科学处理，它无法证明数据来源是否正确。数理统计不能代替科学思维，更不能辩证唯物主义的分析。

Randomization is to divide the subjects into several groups so that they have equal opportunities in the study group and the control group, to minimize the systematic error. Practices that violate the principle of randomization are common in processing studies. For example, after the sample is crushed, it is only one sieve, no upper and lower limits are specified. The animals were grouped first (inactive) into one group and then (lively) into another group. Experimental observation order without randomization and so on. Randomization requires the best efforts of researchers. This is the responsibility of the researcher and also reflects the researcher's scientific research ethics. Why some research results cannot be repeated, although there are many reasons, it has a lot to do with not enough adherence to the principle of randomization.

Repetition is one of the important measures to ensure the reliability of scientific research results. There are two meanings of repetition, one is that the experimental process is repeated many times; the other is that the method and result proposed in the design can be repeated by others. There are reports that rutin in Sophorae Flos (Huaihua) loss a lot after charcoaling, but the content of tanning increased by 4 times, and think that the hemostatic effect of Flos sophorae after charcoal may be due to the increase in tanning. Since then, although there have been some reports that the tanning quantity has not increased, decreased, but further research has proved that the previous report is correct, the study also found that pure rutin can also be converted to tanning after heating, this conversion is closely related to the heating temperature and time. It is not easy to get the reproducibility to result in the processing research, and it is closely related to the heat, time, size and thickness of pieces, extraction condition, and experimental operation technique. The previous thousands of years of processing theory and technology can not be easily denied according to one or two experimental reports.

② **Correct view and selection of mathematical statistics:** There have been two different views on whether to use statistical processing for all kinds of data collected in scientific research. One view holds that mathematical statistics are omnipotent and that they are mysterious; the other holds that mathematical statistics are mathematical games and are skeptical. The proper and correct application of mathematical statistics can bring the data closer to the facts, which is necessary to understand the essence of things.

For example, for someone who uses a certain drug to treat 20 cases of tinea, cure 10 cases, the conclusion is that the cure rate is 50%. This is not credible, and the actual possible range of 10/20 is 27 to 73 percent ($P = 005$) rather than necessarily 50 percent. It can be seen that it is necessary to apply mathematical statistics method properly in processing research, but it must be pointed out that the application of mathematical statistics can only carry out scientific processing of the obtained data, and it cannot prove whether the data source is correct or not. Mathematical statistics cannot replace scientific thinking, let alone dialectical materialism analysis.

炮制研究中得来的测量资料或计数资料常须进行统计学处理，选用的假设检验方法应符合其应用条件。计量资料的比较常用 t 检验，计数资料的比较常用 χ^2 检验，同为计量资料，配对设计与完全随机设计（成组比较）t 检验方法也不相同，如某药材炮制前后实验指标的比较，应为配对资料比较，若用成组比较的 t 检验方法处理，则不但浪费信息，还可能得出错误的结论；同样，不能用大样本的 u 检验代替小样本的 t 检验；也不能用一般的 t 检验代替方差不齐的检验。

The statistical processing of the measured data or counting data obtained from the processing research is often required, and the selected hypothesis test method should meet the application conditions. The method of the t-test is not the same as that of complete random design (group comparison) t-test, for example, the comparison of experimental indexes before and after processing of a medicinal material should be paired data comparison, if we use the t-test method of group comparison, we may not only waste information but also draw the wrong conclusion. Besides, the u-test of the large sample t-test cannot replace the t-test of the small sample, nor the general t-test replaces the test of the uneven variance.

参考文献：

[1] 葛朝亮，刘颖，余剑萍，等.传统中药炮制技术在实验教学中的应用和意义[J].中国中医药现代远程教育，2017，15（03）：23-25.

[2] 董军.张景岳《本草正》中药炮制学术思想探析[J].浙江中医杂志，2021，56（01）：18-19.

[3] 袁国卿.张仲景中药炮制学术思想探析[J].中国中药杂志，2010，35（06）：799-802.

[4] 盛政，赵焕君，何紫涵，等.酒制升提理论的形成发展和临床应用[J].亚太传统医药，2020，16（11）：198-201.

[5] 钟凌云，叶协滔，杨明，等.中药炮制"三适"理论的研究与实践[J].中国实验方剂学杂志，2020，26（10）：180-185.

[6] 唐廷猷.中药炮制理论炮制原理研究史初探（清代前部分）[J].中国现代中药，2018，20（02）：230-238.

[7] 马传江，王信，辛义周，等.中药传统炮制理论的现代研究概述[J].中草药，2018，49（03）：512-520.

[8] 张联.中国药典"炮制通则"中药炮制方法分类探讨[J].中国现代应用药学，

2020, 37 (18): 2287-2290.

[9] 臧慧敏, 焦梦琦, 王美玲, 等. 简谈蒙药的传统炮制方法 [J]. 中国民族医药杂志, 2021, 27 (01): 45-49.

[10] 杨萌, 李超英. 芒硝的炮制历史沿革、炮制方法及临床应用研究进展 [J/OL]. 中药材, 2020 (12): 3069-3074 [2021-05-15].

[11] 甄臻, 王杨, 魏海峰, 等. 基于颜色变化的麸炒山药质量标准及炮制工艺探究 [J]. 中成药, 2021, 43 (03): 816-819.

[12] 阳长明, 杨平, 刘乐环, 等. 中药质量标志物 (Q-Marker) 研究进展及对中药质量研究的思考 [J]. 中草药, 2021, 52 (09): 2519-2526.

[13] 曹雪晓, 任晓亮, 王萌, 等. 中药材及饮片规格等级质量标准研究进展 [J/OL]. 中药材, 2021 (02): 494-498 [2021-05-15].

[14] 高歌, 史相国. 影响中药饮片质量和临床疗效的主要因素及对策 [J]. 中国现代药物应用, 2020, 14 (11): 214-216.

[15] 王蕾, 燕彩云, 乐智勇, 等. 盐制法及炮制辅料盐的炮制历史沿革研究 [J]. 中国中药杂志, 2017, 42 (20): 3880-3885.

[16] 聂黎行, 王钢力, 李志猛, 等. 近红外光谱法在中药辅料质量控制中的应用 [J]. 中国中药杂志, 2009, 34 (17): 2185-2188.

［17］吴萍，张志国，杨磊，等.关于炮制辅料蜜及其炮制品规范的思考［J］.中国现代中药，2020，22（10）：1729-1734.

［18］杨春雨.中药炮制用辅料（姜汁）规范化的探索性研究［D］.北京：中国中医科学院，2018.

［19］汪岩，王月珍，马千里，等.中药炮制炒法及炒制设备研究概况［J］.亚太传统医药，2015，11（24）：64-65.

［20］陈智钦，王一硕，张振凌，等.专利设备炮制熟地黄的工艺研究及成品质量分析［J］.时珍国医国药，2013，24（07）：1641-1643.

［21］贾天柱.中药饮片炮制技术和相关设备研究［J］.中国科技成果，2011，12（11）：61.

［22］曾洁，施晴，臧振中，等.基于全球专利分析的中药制药装备产业技术发展趋势研究［J］.中草药，2020，51（17）：4373-4382.

［23］秦昆明，李伟东，张金连，等.中药制药装备产业现状与发展战略研究［J］.世界科学技术-中医药现代化，2019，21（12）：2671-2677.

［24］李斯楠.对比中药配方颗粒与中药饮片治疗风热感冒的效果研究［J］.中国现代药物应用，2021，15（08）：211-214.

［25］喻录容，侯毅.中药配方颗粒与中药饮片的临床疗效比较［J］.当代

临床医刊，2021，34（02）：96.

［26］孙冬梅.中药配方颗粒和中药饮片临床效果比较［J］.中国中医药现代远程教育，2021，19（06）：36-38.

［27］冯丽.中药配方颗粒省级标准制定关注要点［N］.中国医药报，2021-03-09（003）.

［28］徐玉玲，雷燕莉，曾立，等.中药配方颗粒品种统一标准的有关问题探讨［J］.中草药，2020，51（20）：5389-5394.

［29］李艺博，李娟，刘碧原，等.中药超微粉碎技术应用概况［J］.中华中医药杂志，2020，35（09）：4568-4570.

［30］陈勇军，钱锦花，梁学良，等.中药超微粉均匀性评价研究［J］.中国粉体技术，2014，20（03）：52-55.

［31］刘艳，张振凌，芦锰，等.正交法优选龟甲胶原料龟甲的炮制提取工艺［J］.中国现代中药，2018，20（02）：204-207.

［32］左蕴泽，王卓，周厚江，等.一种龟甲抗肝癌药理作用机制的网络药理学研究［J］.亚太传统医药，2021，17（02）：136-140.

［33］陈铭阳，胡小松，许贞，等.龟甲中具有潜在药理活性的miRNA初步筛选［J］.中国现代中药，2018，20（04）：395-401.

［34］刘斌，陈琴鸣，陈卫平，等.人参芦头多糖的初步研究［J］.中草药，2011，42（12）：2422-2423.

［35］唐开强，穆晓红，叶超，等.乳香-没药治疗类风湿性关节炎的网络药理学和生物信息学分析［J］.世界中医药，2021，16（12）：29-35.

[36] Zwerger M, Ganzera M. Analysis of boswellic acids in dietary supplements containing Indian frankincense (Boswellia serrata) by Supercritical Fluid Chromatography [J]. Journal of Pharmaceutical and Biomedical Analysis, 2021, 201 (2): 114106.

[37] Mv A, Ahd B, Sst D, et al. The effects of Boswellia (Frankincense) gel and hydrocolloid dressing on healing of second-and third-degree pressure ulcers among hospitalized patients [J]. Journal of Herbal Medicine, 2021, 29 (4): 100461.

[38] 赵璇, 李沁, 马彦江, 等. 延胡索醋炙工艺、物性参数及成分含量的相关性研究及回归分析 [J/OL]. 中华中医药学刊: 1-11 [2021-05-15].

[39] Jeong H C, Park J E, Seo Y, et al. Urinary Metabolomic Profiling after Administration of Corydalis Tuber and Pharbitis Seed Extract in Healthy Korean Volunteers [J]. Pharmaceutics, 2021, 13 (4): 522.

[40] 徐超, 林杰, 金传山, 等. HPLC 指纹图谱结合化学计量学比较同株不同生长年限亳白芍化学成分差异 [J]. 中草药, 2021, 52 (08): 2408-2413.

[41] You, G., Li, H., Liu, Y. et al. Comparative Analyses of Radix Paeoniae Alba with Different Appearance Traits and from Different Geographical Origins Using HPLC Fingerprints and Chemossmetrics. Chromatographia, 2020, 83 (12), 1443–1451.

[42] Jia X K, Huang J F, Huang X Q, et al. Alismatis Rhizoma Triterpenes Alleviate High-Fat Diet-Induced Insulin Resistance in Skeletal Muscle of Mice [J]. Evidence-based Complementary and Alternative Medicine, 2021, 2021 (5): 1-15.

[43] Shu P, Yu M, Zhu H, et al. Two new iridoid glycosides from Gardeniae Fructus [J]. Carbohydrate Research, 2021, 501: 108259.

第六章 现代研究主要技术与方法

中药炮制即是将未经加工的生药制成用于不同治疗方法的饮片所采取的一项制药技术。如醋、酒、蜂蜜和食盐水等各种辅料,在炮制过程中可以增强原料药的疗效且降低其毒性。传统上来说,大多数中草药在配药使用前应满足辨证论治的需要,经过适宜的炮制后方能被使用。在确保中药质量与安全性上,炮制起着至关重要的作用。随着中药研究的发展,越来越多的现代技术已经用于中药炮制的现代研究中,比如:①新工艺技术;②代谢组学;③药代动力学;④成分结构理论;⑤分子生物学。

一、新工艺技术的应用

现代中药炮制技术是以现代中药理论为基础,以临床用药和中药制剂相关法律法规为依据。其主要目的是在继承传统中药炮制技术与理论的基础上,遵循中药理论体系,运用现代科学、技术与设备对中药进行加工,使其成品符合饮片质量标准要求且保证药物的安全与有效性。在板蓝根加工过程中产生的废水是中药生产中很重要的一步,而该水是一种有毒且难以处理的废水。Wen Yiyong 等利用离子氧化能够有效分解中药废水中的有机污染物,并且发现在处理过程中可将废水的毒性降低到甚至无毒。实验结果表明,DBD 等离子体技术可能是生物降解中药废水中毒性有机污染物的关键性技术。

第三部分　现代研究

Part III　Modern Research of PCHM

Chapter Six　Main Techniques and Methods of Modern Research of PCHM

PCHM is a pharmaceutical technique that makes raw materials into herbal slices for different therapeutic methods. For instance, all kinds of assistant materials such as vinegar, wine, honey, and brine can enhance the efficacy and reduce the toxicity of crude drugs through processing. Traditionally, most Chinese herbal medicines require proper processing to meet the needs of specific clinical syndromes after being processed. It is the proper processing that plays an essential role in ensuring the quality and safety of TCM[1]. With the development of TCM research, more and more modern technologies have been applied to the modern research of traditional Chinese medicine processing, such as: ① New process technology; ② Metabolomics; ③ Pharmacokinetics; ④ Component Structurology; ⑤ Molecular biology.

Section One　The Application of New Process Technology

Modern Chinese medicine processing technology is based on the theory of modern Chinese medicine, according to the requirements of clinical medication, and relevant laws and regulations of Chinese medicine preparations. It aims to process traditional Chinese medicine by following the theoretical system of traditional Chinese medicine and apply modern science and technology and equipment based on inheriting traditional Chinese medicine processing technology and theory, to make its finished products meet the requirements of quality standards of herbal slices and ensure the safety and effectiveness of the medicine. The wastewater is caused by Isatidis Radix (Banlangeng) processing, which is a type of toxic wastewater and difficult to deal with. Wen Yiyong et al used ionic oxidation to effectively decompose organic pollutants in Chinese medicine wastewater and found that the processing of waste water could reduce its toxicity to a low level or even make it non-toxic. The experimental results show that DBD plasma may be a key technology for biodegradable toxic organic pollutants in traditional Chinese medicine waste-water.

Xue Jintao 等利用近红外光谱法能够快速、同时检测出来自于不同产地、不同炮制方法所处理的大黄中五种主要活性成分（大黄酚、芦荟大黄素、大黄酸、大黄素和大黄素）。并且利用最优 NIR 模型研究区域差异与不同的炮制方法所产生的影响，便于识别假大黄。探究炮制化学是阐述草药传统炮制技术科学理论的关键性步骤，尤其是涉及化学转化机制的时候。

　　Zhou Li 等研究生地黄时提出了创新性的思路，即通过化学组学的标记化合物挖掘和模拟炮制相结合的方法，进而深入研究草药炮制过程中涉及的化学转化机制。通过该方法，能在生地黄与熟地黄中快速的发现一组差异性标志物，包括糖类、糖苷和糠醛。并且地黄在炮制过程中涉及的主要化学机制为经过脱糖转化和/或脱水，逐步转化为糖（多糖、寡糖及单糖）、糖苷（环烯醚萜苷和苯乙醇苷）和糠醛（糖基化/非糖基化羟甲基糠醛）。该研究不但有助于对地黄炮制化学的认识，而且为中草药传统炮制化学研究提供了创新思路。

　　人参中的碳水化合物和人参皂苷在生物学上是相互关联的。因此，它们的同步分析对人参的化学研究至关重要，用以表征其"整体"质量。Xu Jie 等研究发现在红参（即通过蒸法所炮制的人参）的化学炮制过程中，可通过多种分析技术对碳水化合物和人参皂苷进行定性和定量测定。结果表明，蒸制不仅在定性和定量上改变了人参皂苷，而且通过改变生理化学参数影响碳水化合物，即水溶性、分子大小、组成单糖的类型与比例。并且提出、讨论了关于人参制品转化的潜在机制，包括水解（去糖基化、去丙酰化、脱乙酰化）、脱水、聚合、挥发、还原和美拉德反应。该实验强调了红参化学炮制研究，有助于阐明制备和应用的科学依据。

第三部分 现代研究
Part III Modern Research of PCHM

Xue Jintao et al used near-infrared spectroscopy for rapid and simultaneous determination of five main active compositions (chrysophanol, aloe-emodin, rhein, emodin, and physcion) in processed Rhei Radix Et Rhizoma from different geographical origins and used the optimal NIR model to study the geographical area and the impact of processing, identify fake Rhei Radix Et Rhizoma. Exploring processing chemistry, in particular, the involved chemical transformation mechanisms is a key step to elucidate the scientific basis in the traditional processing of herbal medicines.

Studying Rehmanniae Radix (RR, Dihuang), Zhou Li et al put forward a novel strategy, that is, through the combination of chemical group's marker compound mining and simulation processing, the mechanism of chemical transformation involved in the processing of herbal medicine is further studied. By using this strategy, a set of differential marker compounds including saccharides, glycosides, and furfurals in raw and processed RR was rapidly found, and the major chemical mechanisms involved in RR processing were elucidated as stepwise transformations of saccharides (polysaccharides, oligosaccharides, and monosaccharides) and glycosides (iridoid glycosides and phenethylalcohol glycosides) into furfural (glycosylated/non-glycosylated hydroxymethylfurfural) by deglycosylation and/or dehydration. The research indicated that the proposed strategy could deepen the understanding of RR processing chemistry, and provide a novel approach for chemical research in the traditional processing of herbal medicines.

Carbohydrates and ginsenosides in Ginseng Radix Et Rhizoma are biologically interrelated. Their synchronous analysis is therefore essential in chemical research on ginseng to characterize its "holistic" quality. XuJie et al investigated the processing chemistry of Ginseng Radix Et Rhizoma Rubra, and found that a ginseng product processed by water-steaming, for which both carbohydrates and ginsenosides were qualitatively and quantitatively determined through multiple analytical techniques. Results revealed that the stream-processing not only qualitatively and quantitatively altered the ginsenosides but also affected the polymeric carbohydrates *via* changing their physiochemical parameters, *i.e.* water solubility, molecular size, types, and ratios of constituent monosaccharides. Potential mechanisms involved in the transformation of Ginseng Radix Et Rhizoma chemicals are proposed and discussed, including hydrolysis (deglycosylation, decarbonylation, deacetylation), dehydration, polymerization, volatilization, reduction, and the Maillard reaction. The study strengthens the research on the chemical processing of Ginseng Radix Et Rhizoma Rubra and therefore helps throw light on the scientific basis of Ginseng Radix Et Rhizoma Rubra preparation and application.

二、代谢组学

目前，传统炮制机制的研究还不够深入和广泛，过去常用物理化学方法讨论传统炮制机制。研究中药炮制机制是中药炮制学科和中药现代化的关键，代谢组学是后基因组时代的最新发展学科，并将成为中药材料基础研究的重要部分。目前，代谢组学已应用于传统炮制研究。

近几年来，代谢组学技术因其适用于研究复杂系统的完整性而逐渐被引入中药现代化研究，在揭示中药作用机制方面发挥了重要作用。在中药炮制机制研究中，代谢组学方法有助于揭示炮制过程对组分药效学和毒性的影响机制。Zhong Lingyun 等报道以高分辨质谱（HRMS）研究黄连炮制前后对大鼠尿液代谢组学中成分改变的影响。结果表明，黄连经生姜汁炮制后，生物碱含量显著变化，这对能量代谢有显著影响。鉴定了 9 种生物标志物，如肌氨酸、马尿酸和 L- 色氨酸，这些差异产物是由于黄连炮制前后产生了不同的抗炎作用机制引起。

代谢组学方法常用于研究中草药的药理作用和机制。半夏（PR）是一种常用的中草药，但经常有关于其毒性的报道。根据传统中医药理论，炮制可以减少草药的毒性。苏涛等设计了一项研究，以确定炮制是否降低了原料 PR 的毒性，并探讨了原料 PR 引起的毒性的潜在机制和炮制的毒性降低作用。该研究使用生化和组织病理学方法来评估原始和炮制 PR 的毒性，通过 LC-TOF-MS 分析大鼠血清代谢物，代谢组学数据的 Ingenuity 通路分析突出了原始 PR 产生毒性所涉及的生物途径和网络功能以及炮制的毒性降低作用，这些都在分子水平上得到验证。结果表明，原料 PR 引起心脏毒性，炮制降低了毒性。由于半夏原料药诱导的心脏毒性抑制了 mTOR 信号传导并激活 TGF-β 途径，并且清除自由基可能是炮制后毒性降低的原因，数据揭示了原料药 PR 诱导的心脏毒性机制和炮制后毒性降低作用机制。本研究为 PR 的传统炮制理论提供了科学依据，有助于优化炮制方案和半夏的临床联合应用。

第三部分　现代研究
Part III　Modern Research of PCHM

Section Two　Metabolomics

At present, the mechanism of traditional processing is not explored deeply and widely. The chemical and pharmacology methods are mainly used to discuss the mechanism of traditional processing. Study on the mechanism of PCHM is the key to subject of PCHM and modernization of TCM. Metabolomics is a newly developed ascience at the post-genome era and has become an important part of Chinese medicine material basic research. At present, metabolomics has been applied to the study of traditional PCHM.

In recent years, metabolomics technology has been gradually introduced into modern research of TCM because of its applicability to the study of the integrity of complex systems. It has played a very good role in revealing the mechanism of action of TCM. In the study of the processing mechanism of TCM, the metabolomics approach is helpful to reveal the mechanism of the effect of processing products on the pharmacodynamics and toxicity of composition. Zhong Lingyun et al reported that High-resolution mass spectrometry (HRMS) was used to study the effects of composition changes on urine metabonomics of rats before and after processing Coptidis Rhizoma. The results showed that after processing with ginger juice, the contents of alkaloids changed significantly, which had a significant impact on energy metabolism. Nine biomarkers, such as sarcosine, hippuric acid, and L-tryptophan, were identified. These changes were the mechanisms of the difference of anti-inflammatory effects before and after processing Coptidis Rhizoma.

The metabolomics approach is often used to study the pharmacological effect and mechanism of CMM. Pinelliae Rhizoma (PR, Banxia) is a commonly used Chinese medicinal herb, but it has been frequently reported about its toxicity. According to the theory of TCM, processing can reduce the toxicity of the herbs. Su Tao et al designed a study to determine if processing reduces the toxicity of raw PR, and to explore the underlying mechanisms of raw PR-induced toxicities and the toxicity-reducing effect of processing. The study used the biochemical and histopathological approaches to evaluate the toxicities of raw and processed PR. Rat serum metabolites were analyzed by LC-TOF-MS. Ingenuity pathway analysis of the metabolomics data highlighted the biological pathways and network functions involved in raw PR-induced toxicities and the toxicity-reducing effect of processing, which were verified at the level of the molecule. Results showed that raw PR caused cardiotoxicity, and processing reduced the toxicity. Inhibition of mTOR signal and activation of the TGF-β pathway contributed to raw PR-induced cardiotoxicity, and free radical scavenging might be responsible for the toxicity-reducing effect of processing. The data showed new light on the mechanisms of raw PR-induced cardiotoxicity and the toxicity-reducing effect of processing. This study provides scientific justifications for the traditional processing theory of PR and helps to optimize the processing protocol and clinical combinational application of PR.

三、药代动力学

　　Fu zhiling 等以主要成分苦杏仁苷为指标物质,系统地研究了炮制对苦杏仁在大鼠体内的药代动力学过程、组织分布特征以及排泄特征的影响,建立了药材及血浆、组织、尿液样品中苦杏仁苷的 HPLC 分析方法。结果表明,苦杏仁苷在 $0.6 \sim 200\mu g/mL$ 内线性关系良好,高、中、低三个浓度的回收率、日内日间精密度、稳定性等测定结果均符合 FDA 生物样品分析测定的要求,可用于苦杏仁体内作用的研究方法,为炮制影响苦杏仁功效与归经的体内物质基础研究提供了方法学基础。采用上述高效液相色谱的研究方法,对苦杏仁苷单体注射与灌胃给药、苦杏仁生品、焯制品、炒制品、霜制品灌胃给药后在大鼠血浆中的药代动力学过程进行了研究,考察各炮制品与生品及苦杏仁苷单体在大鼠体内代谢过程的差异性。结果表明,灌胃给药后未检测到苦杏仁苷原型,而是产生两个新的代谢产物,经质谱鉴定为野樱苷的同分异构体。并且炮制后野樱苷的药时曲线与生品有明显不同,以霜制的差异最大,出现明显的二次达峰,这为炮制改变苦杏仁的归经研究提供了依据。本研究还对苦杏仁生品及霜制品在大鼠体内的组织分布特征及尿药排泄特征的差异进行了研究,结果表明灌胃给药后可使尿液中的马尿酸含量显著增加,并且霜制后代谢产物野樱苷进入各组织的时间延后,在各时间点的分布量更加平均,使药物在体内的分布时间更长,作用更加持久,为霜制改变苦杏仁的归经提供了一定的参考。

　　Zhao yanhong 等设计了一项实验,在大鼠体内研究了淫羊藿中黄酮类化合物的肠道吸收和代谢,分析比较了淫羊藿中淫羊藿苷和淫羊藿总黄酮的肠道吸收特征差异。药代动力学结果表明,大鼠不同肠段淫羊藿苷单体的吸收特性与淫羊藿总黄酮中的淫羊藿苷吸收特征一致。淫羊藿苷在大鼠不同肠段的吸收存在差异,其中回肠和结肠肠段的可渗透系数明显低于十二指肠和空肠。淫羊藿总黄酮中有多种成分在大鼠肠段会发生代谢转化,其中淫羊藿苷经过大鼠肠段后代谢最为明显。进一步的药理学研究表明,灌胃处理后可以改善淫羊藿中黄酮类化合物的吸收。

Section Three Pharmacokinetics

Fu zhiling et al studied the effects of processing on the pharmacokinetic process, tissue distribution, and excretion characteristics of Armeniacae Semen Amarum (Kuxingren) in rats by taking its main component, amygdalin, as the index substance. They established the first medicine and laetrile in plasma and tissue, urine samples of HPLC analysis method. The results showed that the laetrile in 0.6 ~ 200 μg/mL was good, high, medium, and low three concentration gained recovery precision, stability and days of the determination results are accord with the requirement of the FDA's determination of biological sample analysis, which can provide methodology basis in the research of Armeniacae Semen Amarum in vivo role after processing, the Armeniacae Semen Amarum efficacy and returning to the substance. The high-performance liquid chromatography (HPLC) of laetrile monomer was adopted to inspect raw and processed products and laetrile monomer in rats in vivo metabolic process who had intragastric administration by Armeniacae Semen Amarum, fired products, products processed with oil, cream products to study the pharmacokinetic process. The results showed that no amygdalin prototype was detected after intragastric administration, but two new metabolites were produced, which were identified as isomers of nos by mass spectrometry. Besides, the curve of processing time of wild primrose was different from that of raw product, and the difference was the most obvious in the frosting system, with an obvious secondary peak. The results provide a basis for the processing and transformation of Armeniacae Semen Amarum. In the Armeniacae Semen Amarum and cream products in rats in vivo tissue distribution characteristics and the different characteristics of urine drug excretion were studied, the results show that after gastric drug can make urine hippuric acid content increased significantly, and the frost after metabolites wild cherry glycosides into the time delay of each group at various time points are more evenly, make the distribution of the drug in the body longer, more lasting.

Zhao yanhong et al designed an experiment to study the absorption and metabolism of several monomer chemical compositions such as icariin and total flavonoid extracts in the crystallization and processed products of Epimedii Folium (Yinyanghuo) and tried to elaborate the processing mechanism of icariin from the perspective of effective component of absorption and metabolism. Intestinal absorption and metabolism of flavonoids in Epimedii Folium were investigated in vivo in rats. The differences in intestinal absorption and metabolism of flavonoids in Epimedii Folium and total flavonoids in rats were compared and analyzed. The pharmacokinetic results showed that the absorption characteristics of icariin monomer in different intestinal segments of rats were consistent with that of icariin in total flavonoids in rats. There were differences in the absorption of icariin in different parts of rat intestinal segments, among which the permeability coefficient of ileum and colon intestinal segments was significantly lower than that of duodenum and jejunum. Further pharmacokinetic studies showed that lavage can improve the absorption of flavonoids in Epimedii Folium.

炮制是中药的特色之一，它不仅会改变药物的性质，还会影响药品的质量。然而如何客观有效地评价炮制前后中药质量的变化，是长久以来唯一限制中药发展的瓶颈，也同样困扰着中药质量分析人员。

Zhang yingyue 等根据《中国药典》，分别经过 0、1、2、4 小时炮制杜仲。以马钱子碱（MS）为内标，通过 LC-MS/MS 建立的方法测定不同处理时间杜仲中 4 种目标成分和药代动力学血液成分的含量。实验结果表明，各测定组分各组分的线性关系良好。杜仲的炮制时间应控制在 2 小时内。该研究从体内药代动力学的角度描述了炮制对目标成分的影响，其结果对杜仲的炮制和临床应用具有指导意义。

在中国，生姜（*Zingiber officinale* Rosc.）及其炮制产品，如干姜、炮姜通常在传统中药中应用广泛。Han Y 等研究鲜姜、干姜、炮姜对血瘀证的作用。首先，Han Y 等建立了血瘀证大鼠，然后分析了血液流变学和凝血活性。最后，Han Y 等建立了灵敏、简单、有效的气相色谱结合飞行时间质谱（GC-TOF/MS）方法，结合多变量分析比较代谢指纹图谱。一共有 27 种代谢物（血清 16 种，尿液 11 种）被检出，有助于血瘀证研究。这些代谢产物和不同影响值的 6 种代谢途径有关，有代谢综合征的代谢指标主要涉及不同影响值的 6 种代谢途径，鲜姜（FG）、干姜（D）和炮姜（SG）可将指数和代谢物的变化控制在正常水平。如功效指数，相似性分析和峰强度所示，鲜姜作用效果最明显。结果表明，代谢组学与功效指数结合使得研究血瘀证并且比较鲜姜、干姜、炮姜的作用和代谢产物成为可能。

中药的药代动力学是利用动力学原理和治疗方法定性描述中药的有效成分、有效部位，以及中药通过各种途径进入人体后的吸收、分布、代谢和排泄过程的动态变化。中药的药代动力学在现代中药炮制研究、中医药科研中一直发挥着重要作用。

As one of the characteristics of TCM, PCHM can not only change the property of medicine but also affect its quality. However, how to objectively and effectively evaluate the changes in the quality of Chinese medicine before and after processing is the bottleneck that restricts the development of the processing of Chinese medicine for a long time, as well as the problem that puzzles the quality analysis of Chinese medicine.

Zhang yingyue, et al reported that according to the *Chinese pharmacopeia*, the Eucommiae Cortex (Duzhong) was prepared at 0,1,2, and 4 h, respectively, with strychnine (ms) as internal standard, the contents of four target components and pharmacokinetic hemodynamic components in Eucommia ulmoides were determined by LC-MS/MS. The experimental results show that the linear relationship of each component is good. The processing time of Eucommia ulmoides should be controlled within 2 hours. This study describes the effects of processing on the target components from the perspective of pharmacokinetics in vivo, and its results are instructive to the processing and clinical application of Eucommia ulmoides.

In China, Zingiberis Rhizoma Recens and its processed products, such as Zingiberis Rhizoma and Zingiberis Rhizoma Praeparatum are commonly used in TCM. Han Y et al studied the effects of Zingiberis Rhizoma Recens, Zingiberis Rhizoma, and Zingiberis Rhizoma Praeparatum on blood stasis. First, Han Y et al established a blood stasis syndrome rats model. Then they analyzed the hemorheological and blood coagulation activities. Last, they established a sensitive, simple, and validated gas chromatography combined with the time-of-flight mass spectrometry (GC-TOF/MS) method to compare the metabolic fingerprint coupled with multivariate analysis. A total of 27 metabolites (16 in serum and 11 in urine) were identified, which contributed to the study of blood stasis. These metabolites mainly involve six metabolism pathways in different impact-value. The altered efficacy index and metabolites can be regulated to normal levels by Zingiberis Rhizoma Recens, Zingiberis Rhizoma, and Zingiberis Rhizoma Praeparatum. Zingiberis Rhizoma Recens is the most effective as shown by the efficacy index, similarity analysis, and peak intensity. The result showed that metabolomics equipped with an efficacy index makes it possible to study the blood stasis syndrome and to compare the effect and metabolites in Zingiberis Rhizoma Recens, Zingiberis Rhizoma, and Zingiberis Rhizoma Praeparatum.

By using the principles of kinetics and therapeutic methods, Pharmacokinetics of TCM qualitatively describes the active composition of traditional Chinese medicine, effective parts of CMM, and dynamic Changes of absorption, distribution, metabolism, and excretion of traditional Chinese medicine after it enters the body through various ways. The pharmacokinetics of traditional Chinese medicine has been playing an important role in the processing and scientific research of modern TCM.

从体内暴露水平的角度来看，药代动力学可用于表征体内中药的多组分，总体特征反映了中药在体内主要成分的保留特性，为最终阐明药材炮制对药材治疗效果的影响和建立独特的中医药炮制理论提供了科学依据。

四、组分结构理论

中药炮制学是中医理论体系中最具特色的研究领域之一。中药的物质基础是由多种化学成分组成的，这些化学成分的作用往往是综合作用的结果。

组分结构理论的引入，使现代中药研究更加科学化。通过对中药成分结构的研究，揭示了中药化学成分的组成和应用，从而达到了中药的增效作用，中药疗效是其整体协同作用。中药单体组成是中药最基本的单位，与单体成分按照一定的比例构成成分，并按一定的比例组合成中药整体。这些成分的积累不是简单的，而是一个有序的整体。

有报道，在长期中药成分研究的基础上，研究人员提出了中药配伍理论的组分配伍理论，中药研究的组分配伍理论是以中药理论为指导，根据配伍原则，对特定的疾病适应证，将一些中药组合物根据主效加强，对两个或两个以上弱效，降低配伍原则的副作用，优化设计过程。王琦等研究不同比例川芎嗪和葛根素在偏头痛治疗中的配伍情况，通过测定其血清素等神经递质水平，结果表明，两种中药按4∶3配伍时，配伍效果最好。黄芪及莪术配伍，能显著提高莪术挥发油、莪术烯醇和莪术酮等6个脂溶性成分的溶出率，从而产生协同抗肿瘤作用。

Pharmacokinetics can be used to characterize the multi-component of traditional Chinese medicine in vivo from the perspective of in vivo exposure level. The overall situation reflects the retention characteristics of the main components of traditional Chinese medicine in vivo, which provides a scientific basis for the final clarification of the effects of processing based on CMM and the establishment of a unique theory of PCHM.

Section Four Component Structure Theory

PCHM is one of the most characteristic research fields in the theoretical system of TCM. The material basis of traditional Chinese medicine is composed of a variety of chemical compositions, which often work together to produce an overall effect.

The introduction of the theory of component structure makes modern TCM research more scientific. The study of the composition structure reveals the composition and application of the chemical composition of traditional Chinese medicine, thus achieves the synergistic effect of traditional Chinese medicine. Chinese medicine efficacy is the overall synergy. Monomer composition in traditional Chinese medicine is the most basic unit, which is in a certain proportion of the monomer composition and makes up the Chinese medicine according to a certain proportion of different composition. The accumulation of these compositions is not simple, but orderly as a whole.

It is reported that, based on long-term research on the composition of traditional Chinese medicine, the component compatibility of traditional Chinese medicine theory was put forward by researchers. Composition compatibility of traditional Chinese medicine research is under the guidance of TCM theory. According to the compatibility principle, for specific disease indications, several traditional Chinese medicine compositions strengthen the main effect, with two or more things weak effect, reduces the side effect of compatibility principle, and optimizes design process. Wang Q et al studied the compatibility of ligustrazine and puerarin with different proportions in the treatment of migraines, by measuring the neurotransmitters such as serotonin levels, the results showed that two herbs, ligustrazine, and puerarin works best according to the compatibility of 4:3. The compatibility of Astragali Radix (Huangqi) and Curcumae Rhizoma (Ezhu) can significantly improve the dissolution rate of six fat-soluble compositions of curcuma volatile oil, curcuma enol and curcuma ketone, etc, to produce the synergistic antitumor effect.

在中药炮制研究领域，中药炮制的主要目的包括提高疗效、降低毒性、减轻药物的性质和改变药物作用趋势等。中药炮制过程也可以看作是组分结构或组分配伍变化的过程。目前，它在中药配伍中的应用越来越广泛。半夏与附子有中药配伍禁忌，但附子与半夏配伍的临床应用历史悠久。季延苏等人结果表明，炮制和煎煮均可降低双酯型生物碱的毒性，主要有毒物质经炮制和煎煮后水解后可提高二酯型生物碱的含量。不同炮制方法对双酯型生物碱的水解有不同的抑制作用。因此，采用附子与半夏配伍时，除强调适应证外，还应注意对炮制方法和炮制品种的确定，并辅以附子汤剂以降低毒性。

另外，单味中药在加工过程中会使药物内部物质基础、成分等发生协同衰减，产生结构上的变化，如大黄长大成熟时，结合蒽醌类成分转化为游离蒽醌类成分，使泻下作用减弱，并且抗菌、抗炎、抗肿瘤作用增强。地黄在成熟过程，成分结构发生了显著变化，环烯醚萜类成分的发生水解反应。乌头在炮制过程中，乌头生物碱成分发生了显著变化，双酯型生物碱水解为单酯型生物碱，能显著降低毒性，但其镇痛、抗炎作用保存较好，甚至略有增强。

将组分结构理论应用于中药饮片的研究，有助于揭示中药炮制机制，指导中药饮片的炮制工艺和饮片质量标准的研究，为临床提供高质量的中药饮片。同时，在具体的研究过程中，运用光谱关系和代谢组学的研究思路和方法，有助于揭示中医中药物质基础和机制的作用，为中医研究提供更理想的方法，加快中药现代化研究进程。

Part III Modern Research of PCHM

In the research field of PCHM, Its main purposes include enhancing the effect reducing toxicity, alleviating the property of drugs and changing the tendency of drug action, etc. The process of PCHM can also be regarded as the process of component structure or component compatibility changes. Nowadays, it is more and more widely used in the compatibility of traditional Chinese medicine. Pinelliae Rhizoma (Banxia) and Aconiti Lateralis Radix Praeparata (Fuzi) are incompatibility contraindications of TCM, but the clinical application of the compatibility of Pinelliae Rhizoma and Aconiti Kusnezoffii Radix Lateralis Preparata has a long history. Ji yansu et al showed that processing and decoction could reduce the toxicity of diesteroid alkaloids because the main toxic substances were hydrolyzed after processing and decoction, and the combination of the two drugs could increase the concentration of diesteroid alkaloids. Different processing methods of Pinelliae Rhizoma had different inhibitory effects on the hydrolysis of double ester alkaloids. Therefore, when using the combination of aconite and Pinelliae Rhizoma tuber, in addition to the indications, attention should be paid to the confirmation of the processing of the two drugs, supplemented with aconite decoction to reduce toxicity.

In addition, collaborative attenuation occurs in single Chinese medicine in the process of processing and makes a change in structure. For example, when Rhei Radix Et Rhizoma (Daihuang) grows mature, the combination of anthraquinone components is converted into free anthraquinone components. The effect of diarrhea is weakened, and the antibacterial, anti-inflammatory, and anti-tumor effects of Rhei Radix Et Rhizoma are enhanced. In the mature process of Rehmanniae Radix (Dihuang), the composition structure has undergone significant changes, and the hydrolysis reaction occurs in the components of cycloenedoid. During the processing of aconitum, the composition of aconitine changed significantly, and the hydrolysis of diester alkaloid into monoester alkaloid could significantly reduce the toxicity, but its analgesic and anti-inflammatory effects were well preserved and even slightly enhanced.

A component structure theory was applied to the study of Chinese herbal slices, which helps reveal the mechanism of PCHM, guides the research on processing technology of PCHM and quality standard of Chinese herbal slices, provides high quality of Chinese herbal slices. At the same time, In the specific research process, using the research ideas and methods of spectral relation and metabonomics, it is helpful to reveal the function of TCM material basis and mechanism, to provide a more ideal method for TCM research, and to speed up the research process of TCM modernization.

五、分子生物学技术

目前，以基因工程为主导的生物技术以分子生物学理论为基础，以其强大的生命力，推动着各生命学科的发展。进入 20 世纪 90 年代后，这一高新技术开始在中医药研究领域得到推广和应用。将分子生物学技术引入中药加工中，从基因和分子水平研究中药的基本理论、疾病的性质及中药的作用。这弥补了中医微观还原分析研究的不足，有利于中医从简单的方法论尽快向现代辩证方法的转变。

分子生物学的主要研究对象是生物大分子中的蛋白质和基因核酸。在中药炮制过程中，常常根据药物中蛋白质的变化来说明炮制的效果。陈彦琳等研究了巴豆霜蛋白组分在加工加热前后溶血效果的变化，为巴豆霜的加热脱毒提供依据。本实验通过比较巴豆素在不同加工方法和不同加热时间下的溶血情况，观察其溶血行为。结果发现，加热后巴豆素的溶血作用消失，这与加热时间有关。结论为，巴豆霜的溶血作用的测定可用于控制豆霜的质量。

水蛭是一种具有活血化瘀作用的中药。临床应用主要是以水蛭为主体，由煎煮后的活水蛭经加工而成。有些地区用酒产品，即水蛭切段，加黄酒闷干，慢火炒干。《中国药典》中的水蛭制品是用热滑石粉制成的。上述两种方法都将不可避免地对水蛭进行高温处理。从某种意义上说，水蛭是一个复杂的蛋白质混合系统。高温会破坏蛋白质的空间构象，从而使其失活。因此，为了解水蛭的高温加工是否科学合理，必须在分子生物学领域进行蛋白质分析。Ma Lin 等用现代低温处理方法，即冻干技术对水蛭进行了研究，并对制水蛭和生水蛭进行了相关质量检测和凝血酶活性测定。实验采用 SDS-PAGE 技术探讨水蛭及其炮制品中水溶性蛋白含量的差异，说明高温加工的科学性。结果表明，水蛭中水溶性蛋白的含量在不同加工方法之间存在显著差异，传统的高温处理方法对水蛭中的蛋白质进行了降解，因此，高温加工的科学内涵有待进一步研究。

Section Five Molecular Biology

Nowadays, based on the theory of molecular biology, biotechnology dominated by genetic engineering is promoting the development of various disciplines of life science with its great vitality. After entering the 1990s, this new and high technology began to be popularized and applied in the field of TCM research. Molecular biology technology is introduced into the processing of traditional Chinese medicine to study the basic theory of traditional Chinese medicine, the nature of diseases, and the role of traditional Chinese medicine at the gene and molecular level. This makes up for the deficiency of the study of micro-reduction analysis of TCM, which is beneficial to the transformation of TCM from simple methodology to the modern dialectical method as soon as possible.

The main research object of molecular biology is the protein and gene nucleic acid in biological macromolecules. During PCHM, the effect of processing is often illustrated according to the changes of proteins in drugs. Chen an-lin et al studied the changes of hemolysis effect of defatted Crotonis Semen Pulveratum (Badoushuang) before and after processing, to provide a basis for heating processing detoxification of tiglium. This experiment compared the hemolysis of crotonin in different processing methods and different heating times to observe the hemolysis behavior. It was found that the hemolysis effect of crotonopsin disappeared after heating, which was correlated with the heating time. It is concluded that the hemolytic effect of defatted croton seed powder can be used to control its quality.

Hirudo (Shuizhi) is a kind of traditional Chinese medicine that can promote blood circulation and remove blood stasis. The main clinical application of medical treatment is to take Hirudo as the main body, after frying and boiling, the living Hirudo is processed. Some regions use wine products, that is, cut Hirudo to section, moisten with yellow wine and slowly stir-fry to dry with low heat. The processed Hirudoes in *Chinese pharmacopeia* are made of hot talc powder. Both methods will inevitably process Hirudoes at high temperatures. In a sense, Hirudoes are complex protein mixing systems. High temperature can destroy the spatial conformation of proteins, thus inactivating them. Therefore, to know whether the high-temperature processing of Hirudoes is scientific and reasonable, protein analysis in the field of molecular biology must be carried out. The Hirudoes were studied by Ma Lin et al by using the modern low-temperature treatment method, namely freeze-drying technology, and the related quality and thrombin activity of processed Hirudo and raw Hirudo were measured. The SDS-PAGE technique was used to explore the difference in water-soluble protein content in leeches and their processed products. The results show that the content of water-soluble protein in leech is significantly different among different processing methods, and the traditional high-temperature treatment method has degraded the protein in the leech, so the scientific connotation of high-temperature processing needs further study.

除了蛋白质之外，我们有理由相信，在分子生物学领域中的遗传学在现代中药炮制的研究中也将发挥重要的作用。目前，遗传学的许多应用和对中药功效的研究有关。Ma LingDi 等系统、全面地研究了苦参碱对小鼠体内外 H22 肝癌细胞的抗肿瘤作用，并从免疫学角度探讨苦参碱对机体免疫功能的影响，试图从免疫学角度分析和阐述苦参碱的抗肿瘤作用机制。本研究将小鼠共刺激分子 TIM2 基因导入 H22 细胞，经单克隆稳定筛选，获得了以 TIM2 基因修饰的肝癌细胞瘤苗，以提高肿瘤细胞的免疫原性。从基因的角度进一步了解苦参碱在提高免疫功能方面的作用，将为今后苦参碱加工及其在肿瘤临床治疗中的应用提供有价值的理论基础。

从上面的例子可以看出，一些富含蛋白质的中药在没有分子生物学知识的情况下是无法正确加工炮制的。如何更好地利用分子生物学，是中药炮制加工技术中的一个重要环节。

In addition to protein, it is reasonable to believe that in the future, genetics in the field of molecular biology will also play an important role in the modern study of PCHM. At present, there have been many applications of genetics and studies on the efficacy of traditional Chinese medicine. Ma LingDi et al comprehensively and systematically studied the anti-tumor effects of matrine on mouse H22 liver cancer cells both inside and outside the body, and further discussed the effects of matrine on the immune function of the body, trying to analyze and elaborate the anti-tumor mechanism of matrine from the perspective of immunology. In this study, a new costimulatory molecule TIM2 gene from mice was transferred into H22 cells, and after the monoclonal stable screening, the tumor vaccine of H22 liver cancer cells modified with TIM2 gene was obtained to improve the immunogenicity of tumor cells. The further understanding of matrine's role in improving immune function from the perspective of genes will provide a valuable theoretical basis for future study on matrine processing and its application in the clinical treatment of tumors.

From the above examples, we can know that some protein-rich traditional Chinese medicine cannot be processed well without the knowledge of molecular biology. How to make good use of molecular biology is an important link in the processing technology of TCM.

参考文献：

[1] Wen Y, Yi J, Shen Z, et al. Non-thermal plasma treatment of Radix aconiti wastewater generated by traditional Chinese medicine processing [J]. Journal of Environmental Sciences, 2016, 44 (006): 99-108.

[2] Xue, Jintao, Shi, et al. Near-infrared spectroscopy for rapid and simultaneous determination of five main active components in rhubarb of different geographical origins and processing. [J]. Spectrochimica acta. Part A, Molecular and biomolecular spectroscopy, 2018, 205: 419-427.

[3] 王玉，杨雪，夏鹏飞，等. 大黄化学成分、药理作用研究进展及质量标志物的预测分析 [J]. 中草药, 2019, 50 (19): 4821-4837.

[4] 陈冉，王婷婷，李开铃，等. 免疫调节抗病毒中药的特性与应用 [J]. 中草药, 2020, 51 (06): 1412-1426.

[5] Zhou L, Xu J D, Zhou S S, et al. Chemomics-based marker compounds mining and mimetic processing for exploring chemical mechanisms in traditional processing of herbal medicines, a continuous study on Rehmanniae Radix [J]. Journal of Chromatography A, 2017: S0021967317317016.

［6］Zhong L Y, Su D, Zhu J, et al. Comparison of Coptidis Rhizoma processed with different ginger juice based on metabolomics［J］. China Journal of Chinese Materia Medica, 2016, 41（14）: 2712.

［7］罗林明, 石雅宁, 姜懿纳, 等. 人参抗肿瘤作用的有效成分及其机制研究进展［J］. 中草药, 2017, 48（03）: 582-596.

［8］周琪乐, 徐嵬, 杨秀伟. 中国红参化学成分研究［J］. 中国中药杂志, 2016, 41（02）: 233-249.

［9］Cui M N, Zhong L Y, Zhang D Y, et al. Study progress on Pinelliae Rhizoma processed by replication method［J］. China journal of Chinese Materia Medica, 2020, 45（6）: 1304-1310.

［10］苏涛. 半夏白术天麻汤加减联合依达拉奉治疗急性缺血性脑卒中［J］. 实用中西医结合临床, 2017, 17（12）: 44-45.

［11］李听弦, 张志, 傅敏, 等. 基于能量代谢的姜黄连炮制机制初探［J］. 中草药, 2019, 50（23）: 5785-5789.

［12］邓小燕, 钟凌云, 王婷婷, 等. 不同姜汁制黄连对胃肠功能作用研究［J］. 江西中医药, 2019, 50（02）: 57-61.

［13］Zhiling F U. Effect of processing on metabolism of amygdalin from bitter almond in rat [J]. China journal of Chinese Materia Medica, 2010, 35 (20): 2684.

[14] 袁航, 曹树萍, 陈抒云, 等. 淫羊藿的化学成分及质量控制研究进展 [J]. 中草药, 2014, 45 (24): 3630-3640.

[15] 蒋俊, 崔莉, 孙娥, 等. 基于淫羊藿黄酮类化合物的体内代谢阐述其抗骨质疏松药效物质基础 [J]. 中草药, 2014, 45 (05): 721-729.

[16] 张影月, 韩亚亚, 郝佳, 等. 炮制时间对杜仲指标成分含量及药代动力学影响研究 [J]. 天津中医药大学学报, 2016, 35 (05): 322-326.

[17] Han Y Q, Li Y X, Wang Y Z, et al. Comparison of fresh, dried and stir-frying gingers in decoction with blood stasis syndrome in rats based on a GC-TOF/MS metabolomics approach. [J]. Journal of Pharmaceutical & Biomedical Analysis, 2016, 129: 339-349.

[18] Li Y, Yan H, Han Y, et al. Chemical Characterization and Antioxidant Activities Comparison in Fresh, Dried, Stir-frying and Carbonized ginger [J]. Journal of chromatography. B, Analytical technologies in the biomedical and life sciences, 2016, 1011: 223-232.

[19] 柳献云, 吴颖, 王琦, 等. HPLC测定腰痹通胶囊中盐酸川芎嗪的含量 [J]. 中华中医药学刊, 2012, 30 (02): 425-427.

[20] 魏一萍，王琦，梁春华，等.辛伐他汀和磷酸川芎嗪联合应用对COPD-PH患者6min步行试验效果观察［J］.河北医药，2010，32（07）：805-806.

[21] 姬艳苏，张红霞，邹逸竑.附子与半夏配伍禁忌的研究与思考［J］.江苏中医药，2015，47（04）：55-57.

[22] 梁佳佳，杨丽娜，郑卫华，等.附子炮制及与大黄配伍后酯型生物碱的含量变化研究［J］.世界科学技术-中医药现代化，2014，16（01）：38-44.

[23] 陈彦琳，金峰，杜杰，等.不同制霜方法制备巴豆霜饮片质量比较［J］.中国现代中药，2015，17（11）：1201-1203.

[24] 陈彦琳，杜杰，周林，等.加热炮制对巴豆霜溶血效应影响的初步研究［J］.中国现代中药，2013，15（03）：219-222.

[25] 陈彦琳，杜杰，白宗利，等.十二烷基硫酸钠—聚丙烯酰胺凝胶（SDS）电泳比较加热前后巴豆霜蛋白成分的变化［J］.世界科学技术（中医药现代化），2010，12（06）：948-951.

[26] 欧阳罗丹，胡小松，牛明，等.基于网络药理学的水蛭活血化瘀的作

用机制研究［J］.中国中药杂志，2018，43（09）：1901-1906.

［27］黄秋阳，冷静，甘奇超，等.水蛭及其制剂在心脑血管疾病中的应用［J］.中成药，2019，41（08）：1915-1920.

［28］马莉，马琳，王曙宾，等.动物药水蛭高温炮制的科学合理性［J］.中国中药杂志，2015，40（19）：3894-3898.

［29］Ma L, Ma L, Wang SB, et al. Review on scientific connotation of leech processed under high temperature［J］. China Journal of Chinese Materia Medica. 2015, 40 (19): 3894-3898.

［30］Lingdi Ma, Shihong Wen, Yan Zhan, et al. Anticancer Effects of the Chinese Medicine Matrine on Murine Hepatocellular Carcinoma Cells［J］. Planta Med, 2008, 74 (3): 245-251.

［31］曹建，魏润杰，邓茹芸，等.苦参碱及氧化苦参碱抑制肿瘤作用机制研究进展及展望［J］.中草药，2019，50（03）：753-760.

［32］张明发，沈雅琴.苦参碱抗肝癌药理作用及临床应用的研究进展［J］.药物评价研究，2020，43（01）：157-165.

第七章　对炮制成分和药效变化的现代研究

现代对中药炮制的研究，多集中在炮制工艺、炮制前后成分变化、效应成分等，目的是弄清炮制使药效变化物质基础，揭示炮制变化机制，为临床提供安全可靠的中药饮片药材。但在临床应用上，经常通过炮制来改变药物的性能，达到降低或消除药物毒副作用的目的。减毒增效既是炮制的主要目的，也是现代炮制研究的主要目标。因此，须利用现代分析技术科学、客观地反映炮制前后中药内在化学成分的变化，从而阐明中药炮制的机制，提高临床用药的安全性。随着科学技术的发展，高效液相色谱法（HPLC）、气相色谱法（GC）、质谱法（MS）、超高效液相色谱-串联质谱法（UPLC-MS/MS）等技术手段及代谢组学的研究方法均被应用于检测炮制前后成分的改变，为中药更好地开发和利用提供理论基础。炮制的现代研究主要有以下几个方面。

Chapter Seven   Modern Research on the Changes of Contents and Pharmacological Effects Before and After PCHM

Modern research on PCHM mainly focuses on processing technology, the changes of composition before and after processing, the effective constituents, etc. Its purpose is to clarify the basis of the medicinal effect of the processing changes, reveal the mechanism of the processing changes, and provide safe and reliable herbal slices (decoction pieces) for clinical use. But in the clinical application, the processing is often used to change the properties of drugs, reduce or eliminate the side effects. Reducing toxicity and increasing efficiency is the main purpose of processing and the main goal of modern processing research. Therefore, it is necessary to use modern analytical techniques to objectively reflect the changes of the internal chemical components of herbs (TCM) before and after processing, to clarify the mechanism of processing, and enhance the safety of clinical use. With the development of science and technology, high-performance liquid chromatography (HPLC), gas chromatography (GC), mass spectrometry (MS), UPLC-MS, and other technical means, as well as the research methods of metabolomics, have been applied to detect the changes of constituents before and after processing, providing a theoretical basis for the better development and utilization of traditional Chinese medicine. The main modern PCHM research is as follows.

一、炮制对化学成分变化的影响

1. 炮制对含生物碱类药物的影响

生物碱是一类来源于自然界的含氮有机化合物,具有较复杂的环状结构,氮元素多包含在环内。游离生物碱一般不溶或难溶于水,而易溶于有机溶剂,亦可溶于酸(形成盐)。具有碱性的生物碱多以有机酸盐的形式存在,如柠檬酸盐。少数以无机酸盐的形式存在,如盐酸小檗碱。少数碱性极弱的生物碱以游离态存在,如酰胺类生物碱。无论游离生物碱或其盐类都较易溶于乙醇,所以药物经过酒制后可以提高生物碱的溶出率,从而提高药物的疗效。醋是弱酸,能与游离生物碱结合成盐。生物碱的醋酸盐易溶于水,从而增加水溶液中有效成分的含量。对于亲水性生物碱,在炮制过程中用水洗、水浸等操作时,应尽量减少与水接触的时间,避免生物碱的损失,影响疗效。

2. 炮制对含苷类药物的影响

苷类是糖或糖的衍生物与另一非糖物质(苷元)通过糖的端基碳原子连接而成的一类化合物。苷元的结构差别很大,性质和生物活性上差异很大。一般溶于乙醇或水中,有些苷也易溶于三氯甲烷和乙酸乙酯,但难溶于乙醚和苯。酒作为炮制常用辅料,可提高含苷类药物的溶解度,而增加疗效。大部分苷类成分易溶于水,故中药在炮制过程中用水处理时应少泡多润,以免苷类成分溶于水而流失,或发生水解而消失。苷类成分常与酶共存于植物体中,在一定温度和湿度条件下苷可被相应的酶分解,从而使含量减少而降低或失去疗效。所以含苷类药物常用炒、蒸、烘、或暴晒的方法破坏或抑制酶的活性,以免有效成分被酶解。

Part III Modern Research of PCHM

Section One   Effect on the Changes of Chemical Composition by Processing

1. Effects of processing on drugs containing alkaloid

Alkaloids are a kind of nitrogenous organic compounds that come from nature and have a complex ring structure. Nitrogen is mostly contained in the ring. Free alkaloids are generally insoluble in water or hard to dissolve in water, but soluble in organic solvents and soluble in acid water (forming salts). Alkaloids with alkalinity are mostly in the form of organic salts, such as citrate. A few with very weak alkalinity are inorganic salt either, such as amide alkaloids. A few are in the form of inorganic salts, such as berberine hydrochloride. Both free alkaloids and their salts are more soluble in wine. Therefore, the dissolution rate of alkaloids can be improved after processing drugs with wine, thus improving the efficacy of drugs. Vinegar is a weak acid and can combine with free alkaloids to form a salt. The acetate of alkaloids is easily dissolved by water, thus increasing the content of active components in an aqueous solution. For drug-containing hydrophilic alkaloids, the operation of water washing and water immersion in the processing process should minimize the time of contact with water, avoid the loss of alkaloids, to affect the curative effect.

2. Effects of processing on drugs containing glycoside

Glycosides are compounds which are formed when a derivative of sugar or sugar is linked to another non-sugar substance (aglycone) by carbon atoms at the end of sugar. the structure of the glycosides is very different, and the properties and biological activities are very different. Generally soluble in ethanol or water, some glycosides are also soluble in chloroform and ethyl acetate but are insoluble in ether and benzene. As a common excipient, wine can improve the solubility of glycosides and increase the curative effect. Most of the glycosides are soluble in water, so traditional Chinese medicine should be treated with less foam and more moisturizing in the process of processing, to avoid the loss of the glycosides from soluble in water or the occurrence of hydrolysis to disappear. Glycosides often coexist with enzymes in plants. They can be decomposed by corresponding enzymes under certain temperature and humidity conditions, thus reducing the content and reducing or losing the curative effect. Therefore, drugs containing glycoside are commonly processed with stir-frying, steaming, baking, or exposure to the sun to destroy or inhibit the activity of enzymes, lest the active components are enzymatically hydrolyzed.

3. 炮制对含挥发油类药物的影响

挥发油具有挥发性，可随水蒸气蒸馏，与水不相混溶，为油状液体；一般具有芳香性，常温下可自行挥发且不留痕迹，大多数比水轻，溶于多种有机溶剂及脂肪油中，可全溶于 70% 的乙醇中。游离状态的挥发油在自然状态下易于挥发损失，所以像薄荷、荆芥等宜在采收后或喷润后迅速加工切制，不宜带水堆积久放，以免挥发油损失，影响质量。有些药物须要通过炮制以减少或除去挥发油。药物经炮制后，不仅使挥发油的含量发生变化，也使其发生质的变化，如颜色加深、折光率增大，或产生新的成分，有的还可改变药理作用。

4. 炮制对含鞣质类药物的影响

鞣质是由没食子酸（或其聚合物）的葡萄糖（及其他多元醇）酯、黄烷醇及其衍生物的聚合物及两者混合共同组成的植物多元酚。可分为水解鞣质、缩合鞣质、符合鞣质三大类。极性较强，易溶于水，尤其是热水。鞣质为强还原剂，暴露于日光和空气中易被氧化，颜色加深，在碱性溶液中变色更快，所以在炮制过程当中要特别注意。鞣质能耐高温，经高温炮制处理，一般变化不大。鞣质遇铁能发生化学反应，生成墨绿色的鞣质铁盐沉淀，影响中药的外观和内在品质，因而在炮制含鞣质成分的药物时，应避免鞣质与铁反应。

5. 炮制对含有机酸类药物的影响

有机酸类分子结构中含有羧基，在植物中广泛分布，特别是未成熟的肉质果实内。一般与钾、钠、钙、镁、镍、钡等离子结合成盐类存在，有些与生物碱类结合成盐；脂肪酸多与甘油结合成酯或与高级醇结合成蜡；有些有机酸是挥发油与树脂的组成成分。因此，在炮制时用水处理时宜采用少泡多润的方法，以防止有机酸类成分的损失。

3. Effects of processing on drugs containing volatile oils

Volatile oil, an oily liquid, is volatile and can be distilled with water vapor and not miscible with water. Generally, it can be self-volatilization without leaving a trace at room temperature, lighter than water, soluble in a variety of organic solvents and fat oil, and completely soluble in 70% of ethanol. Free state volatile oil in the natural state is easy to volatilize, so herbs, like Menthae Haplocalycis Herba (Bohe), Schizonepetae Herba (Jingjie), should be processed quickly after collecting and spraying, and should not be stacked for a long time so as not to volatilize and thus affect quality. Some medicines should be processed to reduce or remove volatile oils. After the processing of drugs, not only the content of volatile oil changes, but also its qualitative changes, such as color deepening, increased refractive index, or the production of new components, some can also change pharmacological effects.

4. Effects of processing on drugs containing tannins

Tannins are plant polyphenols consisting of a mixture of gallic acid (or its polymer), glucose (and other polyols) esters, flavanols and their derivatives, and a mixture of the two. It can be divided into three categories: hydrolyzed tanning, condensed tanning, and conforming tanning. Its polarity is strong and it is soluble in water, especially hot water. As a strong reducing agent, tannins are easy to be oxidized when it is exposed to sunlight and air, the color is deepened and faster discoloration even occurs fast in alkaline solution. so special attention must be paid to the process of processing. Tannins can withstand high temperatures and there is almost no change after high-temperature processing. Tannins can react with iron to produce dark green tannin iron salt precipitation, which affects the appearance and inner quality of Chinese traditional medicine. Therefore, the reaction between tannins and iron should be avoided when processing drugs containing tannins.

5. Effects of processing on drugs containing organic acids

Organic acids contain carboxyl groups and are widely distributed in plants, especially in immature fleshy fruits. Generally, they can bind to salts with potassium, sodium, calcium, magnesium, nickel, barium plasma, and sometimes bind to salts with alkaloids. Fatty acids combine with glycerol to form ester or with high alcohol to form wax. Some organic acids are constituents of volatile oils and resins. Therefore, they should be processed with a short soak and more moisture in water during processing to prevent the loss of organic acids.

6. 炮制对含油脂类药物的影响

油脂主要成分为长链脂肪酸的甘油酯，大多存在于植物的种子中，通常具有润肠通便或致泻等作用，有的作用峻烈，有一定的毒性。对于含毒性油脂的中药，炮制过程中，经加热、压榨除去部分油脂类成分，以免滑肠致泻或降低毒副作用，保证临床用药安全。如柏子仁制霜，减少部分脂肪油，降低或消除了滑肠作用；千金子去油制霜以减小毒性，使药力缓和。

7. 炮制对含树脂类药物的影响

树脂大多数是由萜类化合物在植物体内氧化、聚合而生成的，通常存在于植物组织中的树脂道中，与挥发油共存的称油树脂（如松油脂），与树胶共存的称胶树脂（如阿魏），与芳香族有机酸共存的称香树脂（如安息香）。树脂多有一定的生理活性，具有防腐、祛痰、消炎、镇静、镇痛、解痉、活血、止痛等作用。炮制可增强某些含树脂类药物的疗效，如乳香、没药醋制后，能增强活血止痛作用，但加热不当，可促使树脂变性，反而会影响疗效。

8. 炮制对蛋白质、氨基酸类药物的影响

蛋白质是一类大分子的胶体物质，多数可溶于水，生成胶体溶液，一般煮沸后由于蛋白质凝固则不再溶于水。所以，含有此类成分的药材不宜长期浸泡于水，以免损失有效成分，影响疗效。炮制时加热可使蛋白质凝固变性，大多数氨基酸遇热亦不稳定。所以，某些富含蛋白质、氨基酸类药效成分的药材以生品为宜，如天花粉、蜂毒等。一些含有毒性蛋白质的中药可通过加热处理，使蛋白质变性从而降低或消除毒性。蛋白质能与许多蛋白质沉淀剂（如鞣质、重金属盐等）产生沉淀，因此，一般不宜和鞣质类的药材一起加工炮制。

6. Effects of processing on drugs containing lipid

The main component of grease is the glyceride of long-chain fatty acid, which mostly exists in the seeds of plants, and usually has the effect of loosening the bowel to relieve constipation or causing diarrhea, and some have severe effects and have certain toxicity. For traditional Chinese medicine containing toxic oil, during the processing, part of the oil components are removed by heating and pressing, to avoid diarrhea caused by the slippery intestine, or reduce the toxic and side effects, to ensure the safety of a clinical medication. For instance, the frost-like powder of Platycladi Semen (Baiziren) is made to reduce part of the fat oil to reduce or eliminate the effect of slippery bowel, the frost-like powder of Euphorbiae Semen (Qianjinzi) is made to reduce toxicity and moderate the drug efficacy.

7. Effects of processing on drugs containing resinous

Resins are mostly formed by the oxidation and polymerization of terpenoids in plants, usually exist in the resin canal of plant tissue. Coexisting with volatile oil is an oleoresin (e.g. pine oil), coexisting with gum is gum resin (e.g. Ferulae Resina), and coexisting with aromatic organic acids is aromatic resin (e.g. Benzoinum). They have certain physiological activity and have the function of anticorrosive, expectorant, and anti-inflammatory, sedative, and analgesic, spasmolysis, activating blood, relieving pain, etc. Processing can enhance certain curative effects of some drugs containing resinous. For example, processing Olibanum (Ruxiang) and Myrrh with vinegar, the effects of the circulation of blood and relieve the pain of drugs can be invigorated. However, improper heating can promote resin degeneration, thus affect efficacy.

8. Effects of processing on drugs containing protein and amino acid

Protein is a kind of colloidal material with large molecules, most of which can be soluble in water to generate a colloidal solution, generally after boiling the protein solidified are no longer soluble in water. Therefore, the medicinal materials containing this kind of ingredients should not be soaked in water for a long time, so as not to lose the effective components and affect the curative effect. During processing, heating can coagulate and denature proteins, and most amino acids are unstable when heated. Therefore, Some medicinal materials rich in protein and amino acids are suitable for use in raw materials, such as Trichosanthis Radix (Tianhuafen) and bee venom (Fengdu). Some traditional Chinese medicines containing toxic proteins can be heated to denature the proteins and reduce or eliminate the toxicity. Protein can precipitate with many protein precipitators (such as tannins, heavy metal salts, etc.), so it is generally not suitable for being processed with drugs containing tannins.

9. 炮制对含糖类药物的影响

糖类可分为单糖、低聚糖和多糖。单糖及小分子寡糖易溶于水，在热水中溶解度更大。多糖难溶于水，但能被水解成寡糖、单糖。因此，在炮制含糖类成分的药物时，一般应尽量少用水处理，必须用水浸泡时要少泡多润，尤其注意与水共同加热的处理。糖和苷元可结合成苷，故一些含糖苷类药物在加热处理后，可分解出糖。

10. 炮制对含无机化合物类药物的影响

无机化合物大量存在于矿物、动植物化石和甲壳类药物中，在植物药中也含有较多的无机盐类，如钠、钾、钙、镁盐等，大多与组织细胞中的有机酸结合成盐而存在。炮制矿物类药物通常采用煅烧或煅烧醋淬的方法，除了可改变其物理性状、使之易于粉碎、有利于有效成分溶出外，也有利于药物在胃肠道的吸收，从而增加疗效。某些含结晶水的矿物药，经煅制后失去结晶水而改变药效。有的药物中所含无机成分在加热后可转化为有毒物质或增加有害物质，如朱砂受热会增加游离汞含量，使毒性增强，此类矿物药应避免受热。

二、炮制对中药药理作用的影响

1. 降低毒性

中药的治疗作用其实就是药物的偏性，也是药物治疗疾病的性能。中药炮制解毒对于其临床使用具有深远的意义。利用高效液相色谱法、代谢组学等分析技术可以客观、科学地研究中药炮制的减毒作用，更好地服务于临床安全用药。如通过 HPLC-MS 方法分别测定芫花炮制前后 5 种化学成分，发现芫花经炮制后，其主要毒副作用成分芫花酯甲含量降低，从而达到了减毒的作用。现代研究表明，可借助仪器分析技术，以探讨中药炮制前后毒性成分变化情况。

9. Effects of processing on drugs containing saccharides

Saccharides can be divided into monosaccharides, oligosaccharides, and polysaccharides. Monosaccharides and small molecule oligosaccharides are easily soluble in water and more soluble in hot water. Polysaccharide is difficult to dissolve in water but can be hydrolyzed into oligosaccharides and monosaccharides. Accordingly, in the processing of drugs containing saccharides, they should be processed with as little water as possible, with a short soak and more moisture time in the water during processing, special attention should be paid during processing with heat and water together. Sugar and aglycone can be combined to form glycosides, so some drugs containing glycosides can be decomposed into sugars after being heated.

10. Effects of processing on drugs containing inorganic compounds

Inorganic compounds exist in a large number of minerals, animal and plant fossils, and crustaceans. Inorganic salts, such as sodium, potassium, calcium, and magnesium salts, are also found in plant drugs. Most of them combine with organic acids in tissue cells to form salts. Processing mineral drugs usually use calcining or calcining with vinegar quenching method, which changes drugs' physical properties and makes them easy to crush, it is beneficial to the dissolution of active components and the absorption of drugs in the gastrointestinal tract, thus increasing the curative effect. Some mineral drugs containing crystal water change their efficacy after calcining. The inorganic composition in some drugs can be converted into toxic material or increase harmful material after heating, for instance, if heating Cinnabaris (Zhusha), the content of free mercuric will increase the toxicity is enhanced, such mineral drugs should avoid heating.

Section Twenty   Effect of Processing on Pharmacological Action of Traditional Chinese Medicine

1. Reducing toxicity

The therapeutic effect of reducing the toxicity of traditional Chinese medicine is the bias of drugs and the performance of drugs to treat diseases. The detoxification of PCHM has far-reaching significance for its clinical use. High-performance liquid chromatography, metabolomics, and other analytical techniques can be used to objectively and scientifically study the toxicity reduction effect of PCHM, to better serve the drugs' clinical safety use. For example, HPLC, MS method was used to determine the 5 chemical constituents of Genkwa Flos (Yuanhua) before and after processing. It was found that the main component of Yuanhuacine with side effects decreased after processing, thereby reducing toxicity. In modern research, the changes of toxic components before and after processing traditional Chinese medicine can be studied through instrumental analysis.

2. 增强药物疗效

现代研究表明，中药通过适当炮制后，可增强药物疗效。如通过 GC-MS 分析发现肉豆蔻经炮制后挥发油成分发生了质和量的变化，其中止泻成分甲基丁香酚、甲基异丁香酚含量增加，而毒性成分肉豆蔻醚、黄樟醚含量降低，从而达到增效减毒的目的。此外，在对比山茱萸炮制前后化学成分变化发现，山茱萸经酒蒸制后，尽管多糖含量下降，但炮制可能改变了多糖的化学组成和结构，所以反而增强其补益肝肾的作用。

3. 药性改变

由于中药中含有多种化学成分，也具有多种药理作用，但治病过程中并不是所有的作用都是有效的。因此，通过炮制"制其性"，也就是说通过使用一些辅料去改变中药的药性，改变中药内在的化学成分，增强或减弱药物的某种或某些药效。在炮制具有典型寒热药性的药物时，通过"以热制寒""以寒制热"，或者使"寒者益寒""热者益热"，扶其不足，增强药性。如生黄连苦寒之性颇盛，善清心火，经胆汁炒后其寒性增加，可以去肝胆实火等。清蒸或用酒炙地黄后，生地黄药性由凉转温，可用于治疗月经不调、肝肾阴亏等证。采用色谱技术，对地黄生熟前后的化学成分进行了对比，结果发现生地黄中含有的多量成分梓醇含量降低，5-羟甲基糠醛（5-HMF）的含量升高。梓醇具有缓泻作用，是生地黄表现凉性的主要成分之一，而 5-HMF 可增加红细胞在毛细血管中流动时的变形性，提高红细胞的通过能力，因而具有活血、补血的作用，是熟地黄表现温性的活性成分之一，进一步验证了炮制后地黄药性由寒变温。

现代研究对中药炮制前后的化学成分和药理作用等变化观察，能为发生炮制变化的药效物质基础提供科学研究的数据支撑，以便深入阐述炮制作用机制，更好地服务于临床。

2. Enhance drug efficacy

Modern research shows that traditional Chinese medicine can enhance the curative effect after proper processing. For instance, GC. MS analysis showed that the content of essential oil of Myristicae Semen (Roudoukou) changed in quality and quantity after processing, among which the content of anti-diarrhea components methyl eugenol and methyl isoeugenol increased, while the content of toxic components nutmeg ether and safrole ether decreased, to achieve the purpose of enhancing effect and reducing toxicity. In addition, after comparing the changes of chemical composition before and after processing of Corni Fructus (Shanzhuyu), Despite the decrease of polysaccharide content after the drug being processed with wine steaming, the processing may change the chemical composition and structure of polysaccharide, so the effect of tonifying liver and kidney was enhanced.

3. Changes drug properties

Though there are many chemical components and pharmacological effects in traditional Chinese medicine, not all of them are effective in curing diseases. Accordingly, the processing is to "change drug properties", that is to say, that says, by using some assistant materials, to change the properties of traditional Chinese medicine, to change the internal chemical composition of traditional Chinese medicine, to enhance or weaken some of the efficacy of the drug. In the processing of drugs with typical cold and heat properties, through 'making cold with heat', 'making heat with cold', or making 'cold even colder', 'hot even hotter, to help its deficiency and enhance its properties. For example, the effect of raw product of Goptidis Rhizoma (Huanglian) with properties of cold and bitter is to clear heart fire, after being processed with bile, the cold property is enhanced, and the effect changes to remove excessive heat of liver and gallbladder. After steaming or stir-frying with wine, the property of unprocessed Rehmanniae Radix (Shengdihuang) changes from cool to warm, it can be used to treat irregular menstruation, liver, and kidney Yin deficiency, and other syndromes. The chemical composition of Rehmanniae Radix before and after processing was compared by chromatography. The results showed that the content of catapol in Rehmannia root decreased, and the content of 5-HMF increased. Catapol has the function of relieving diarrhea and is one of the main components of the coolness of the drug, while 5-HMF can increase the deformability of the red blood cells in the capillary flow and improve the passing ability of the red blood cells, thus it has the function of activating blood and tonifying blood, and it is one of the active components of the warmness of prepared Rehmanniae Radix, which further verified that after processing, that is, the property of Rehmanniae Radix changed from cool to warm.

Modern research on the changes of chemical composition and pharmacological action before and after processing of traditional Chinese medicine can provide the data support for scientific research based on pharmacodynamic substances of processing changes, to expound the mechanism of processing action and better serve the clinic.

参考文献：

[1] 孙娥，徐凤娟，张振海，等.中药炮制机制研究进展及研究思路探讨[J].中国中药杂志，2014，39（03）：363-369.

[2] 李聪，刘红宁，陈丽华，等.加工技术对中药挥发油成分差异性分析[J].中国新药杂志，2021，30（06）：520-527.

[3] 于现阔，吴宏伟，罗寒燕，等.盐炙对沙苑子中沙苑子苷A、B在大鼠体内的药代动力学影响研究[J/OL].中国中药杂志：1-7[2021-07-20].https：//doi.org/10.19540/j.cnki.cjcmm.20210304.301.

[4] 陈君君，蒋志勇.中药炮制对含苷类药物有效性及安全性的影响[J].临床合理用药杂志，2021，14（04）：126-127.

[5] Tian Q，Zhou W，Cai Q，et al. Concepts, processing, and recent developments in encapsulating essential oils[J]. Chinese Journal of Chemical Engineering，2021（2）：255-271.

[6] Akiba Shuichiro, Sahashi Yoshiro, Mitsuma Tadamichi. Effect of heat processing on the quality and alkaloid contents of Coptis Rhizome[J]. Traditional & Kampo Medicine，2020，8（1）：49-54.

[7] 刘睿，刘逊，赵明，等.基于"蛋白质组-修饰组"研究砂炒炮制对穿

山甲蛋白质类成分的影响［J］.中草药，2020，51（13）：3416-3423.

［8］张晶.基于药代动力学研究大黄生、熟饮片的向位药性差异［D］.北京：中国中医科学院，2020.

［9］Cui Wu, Liang Xu, Bo Xu. Correlation between 5-hydroxymethylfurfural content and color of Rehmanniae Radix and Rehmanniae Radix Praeparata［J］. Journal of Chinese Pharmaceutical Sciences，2020，29（05）：314-321.

［10］王丽.何首乌炮制后化学成分及药理作用分析［J］.中国现代药物应用，2020，14（06）：229-231.

［11］邢娜，彭东辉，张志宏，等.炮制对三七化学成分及药理作用影响的研究进展［J］.中国实验方剂学杂志，2020，26（16）：210-217.

［12］苏曼，陈军，高洁，等.生姜炮制成干姜前后挥发油透皮吸收促进作用的比较研究［J］.中草药，2019，50（24）：5988-5994.

［13］钟凌云，崔美娜，杨明，等.炮制影响中药药性的现代研究［J］.中国中药杂志，2019，44（23）：5109-5113.

［14］周园，董秋菊，周玲玉，等.大菟丝子及其清炒品中黄酮和有机酸类成分含量的比较［J］.时珍国医国药，2019，30（09）：2131-2133.

［15］刘亮镜，徐斌，张强.白芍炮制过程中的美拉德反应及芍药苷的变化

［J］. 中华中医药学刊，2020，38（03）：74-77+264.

［16］李新华，李占芳. 中药炮制对药性和临床疗效的影响［J］. 中国中医药现代远程教育，2019，17（12）：49-50.

［17］贾天柱. 中药炮制药性变化论［J］. 中成药，2019，41（02）：470-471.

［18］曾艳，钟为群. 中药炮制对含苷类药物疗效及毒副作用的影响［J］. 中国中医药现代远程教育，2019，17（02）：54-56.

［19］Shan X L, Yu H L, Wu H, et al. Intestinal toxicity of different processed products of Crotonis Fructus and effect of processing on fatty oil and total protein［J］. China journal of Chinese Materia Medica，2018，43（23）：4652-4658.

［20］杨冰，秦昆明，徐滢，等. 决明子生品及炮制品中无机元素的含量测定［J］. 中华中医药杂志，2018，33（08）：3294-3299.

［21］苏松柏，张丽丽，朱迪，等. "九蒸九晒"与《中国药典》两种炮制方法对黑芝麻中氨基酸成分的影响规律研究［J］. 时珍国医国药，2018，29（07）：1631-1633.

［22］刘鹏，孙美玲，李淑军，等. 炮制对黑芝麻油脂的理化性质及润肠通便作用的影响［J］. 特产研究，2017，39（04）：17-20.

[23] 王卫, 王奎龙, 单雪莲, 等. 有毒中药的炮制解毒技术及共性解毒机制 [J]. 南京中医药大学学报, 2017, 33 (05): 448-462.

[24] 万立夏. 中药炮制和用法对药物作用的影响研究 [J]. 中国医药指南, 2017, 15 (24): 190-191.

[25] 蔡琳, 沈美玲. 不同炮制方法对山楂 pH 值及有机酸含量变化的研究 [J]. 山东化工, 2017, 46 (16): 34-35.

[26] 胡梦, 王瑞生, 文雯, 等. 百药煎传统炮制过程中微生物的分离与初步鉴定及其鞣质水解能力测定 [J]. 中国现代中药, 2017, 19 (08): 1120-1125.

[27] 张冰, 林志健, 张晓朦. 基于"识毒-用毒-防毒-解毒"实践的中药药物警戒思想 [J]. 中国中药杂志, 2017, 42 (10): 2017-2020.

[28] 袁海建, 贾晓斌, 印文静, 等. 炮制对半夏毒性成分影响及解毒机制研究报道分析 [J]. 中国中药杂志, 2016, 41 (23): 4462-4468.

[29] 徐莹. 僵蚕炮制前后蛋白质的差异研究 [D]. 镇江: 江苏大学, 2016.

[30] Ebere C.O & Emelike N.J.T. Influence of Processing Methods on the Tannin Content and Quality Characteristics of Cashew By-Products. Agriculture and Food Sciences Research, Asian Online Journal Publishing Group, 2015, 2 (2): 56-61.

[31] 盛菲亚, 卢君蓉, 彭伟, 等. 香附炮制前后挥发油的 GC-MS 指纹图谱

对比研究[J].中草药,2013,44(23):3321-3327.

[32]黄琪,孟江,吴德玲,等.黄芩炒炭前后鞣质含量及炭素吸附力的比较[J].中国实验方剂学杂志,2013,19(22):82-84.

[33]李林,关洪月,殷放宙,等.HPLC-MS测定芫花炮制前后5种成分含量变化[J].中国实验方剂学杂志,2013,19(24):66-70.

[34]刘帅,李飞,侯跃飞,等.诃子中的鞣质成分对诃子汤制草乌的影响——诃子制草乌炮制原理探讨Ⅰ[J].中国实验方剂学杂志,2013,19(05):158-160.

[35]王光宁,杨银凤,陈秋兰.木瓜不同炮制品中水溶性有机酸的含量比较[J].中国现代药物应用,2012,6(22):5-6.

[36]郭东艳,师延琼,王幸,等.大黄不同炮制品中鞣质含量的测定[J].现代中医药,2012,32(04):76-78.

[37]王艳杰,董欣,刘晓波,等.斑蝥炮制前后蛋白质及氨基酸含量测定[J].吉林中医药,2010,30(10):904-905.

[38] 白宗利, 王岩, 贾天柱. 柴胡醋制前后挥发油成分的GC-MS分析 [J]. 中成药, 2009, 31 (09): 1397-1398.

[39] 王伽伯, 马永刚, 张萍, 等. 炮制对大黄化学成分和肝肾毒性的影响及其典型相关分析 [J]. 药学学报, 2009, 44 (08): 885-890.

[40] 李景丽, 袁武会, 于坚, 等. 乌梅制炭前后有机酸和鞣质的含量变化 [J]. 时珍国医国药, 2009, 20 (01): 63-64.

[41] 丁霞, 朱方石, 余宗亮, 等. 山茱萸炮制前后宏微量元素及氨基酸成分比较研究 [J]. 中药材, 2007 (04): 396-399.

[42] 袁子民, 王静, 吕佳, 等. 肉豆蔻饮片炮制前后挥发油成分的GC-MS分析 [J]. 中国中药杂志, 2006 (09): 737-739.

[43] 蔡立明. 乳香等含挥发油树脂类中药炮制方法改进 [J]. 时珍国医国药, 2000 (04): 304.

[44] 程一平. 中药炮制对中药饮片的化学成分及疗效影响研究 [J]. 内蒙古中医药, 2017, 36 (20): 81.

第八章　研究实例

本章选取了目前研究较为成熟的十五个炮制领域研究实例，对目前围绕传统炮制技术所开展的现代技术研究，如炮制工艺的规范与优化、饮片质量标准的测定与制定、饮片炮制机制的阐明等，都进行了概要性描述，以期为今后从事中药炮制科学研究提供有益的思路和线索。

实例一　青黛炮制过程各环节原理的系统研究

研究通过分析历代本草典籍中青黛的炮制方法，结合现代炮制经验和国外制靛染布工艺，采用 HPLC-ELSD、pNPG、SEM 等科学方法和 Plackett-Burman、Box-Behnken 统计学方法，从浸泡、粗靛制备、水飞精制等环节，对中间及最终产物进行定性定量分析。①传统浸泡环节：吲哚苷从马蓝茎叶中释放出来溶解于水中，同时伴随着 β-葡萄糖苷酶催化水解的过程。②粗靛制备环节：将传统的一步制靛分为靛合成和靛分离两步，即用 $NH_3 \cdot H_2O$ 代替石灰，调节氧化反应所需 pH 值，石灰仅作为靛蓝、靛玉红顺利沉降的载体，减少石灰用量。③水飞精制环节：靛蓝、靛玉红与粗靛混悬体系中的蛋白质或多肽等表面活性物质通过非特异性吸附而被分离。④物质变化：吲哚苷经酶解生成吲哚酚，其在有氧条件下生成吲哚酚自由基，一分子吲哚酚自由基与一分子吲哚酚缩合成一分子靛白，其在有氧条件下形成靛蓝；若吲哚酚自由基进一步氧化成为吲哚满二酮，一分子吲哚满二酮与一分子吲哚酚形成靛玉红。⑤炮制工艺：系统地研究了影响青黛炮制过程的因素，分别优化得出定向生成靛蓝、靛玉红的两条工艺路线。以上研究，为建立青黛饮片炮制的规范化、可控化、产业化奠定了基础。

（引自江西中医药大学杨明主持的国家自然科学基金项目"青黛炮制过程各环节原理的系统研究"；项目编号：30772784）

第三部分 现代研究

Part III Modern Research of PCHM

Chapter Eight Examples of Modern Research of PCHM

Fifteen examples of research in the processing field are chosen to provide beneficial thoughts and clues. The modern technical research in traditional processing, such as the normative and optimization of processing process, formulation of qualify bastardization of pieces or slices, and clarification of processing mechanism are generally described in this chapter.

Example 1 Systematical Research of Processing Mechanism During Every Step in Processing of Indigo Naturalis

According to the record of processing of Indigo Naturalis in ancient medical books, combing with modern processing experience and abroad process of making indigo cloth, in the steps of soaking, crude preparation and levigating to refine powder with water, HPLC-ELSD、pNPG、SEM and Plackett-Burman、Box-Behnken were applied to analyze the qualitative and quantitative of the intermediate and final product of Indigo Naturalis. Step 1: Traditional soaking Ndole glycoside is resolved in water from stem and leaf of Strobilanthes cusia, combining with the hydrolysis of β-glucosidase. Step 2: Preparation of crude indigo The traditional preparation is separated into indigo synthesis and indigo separation, which means to use $NH_3 \cdot H_2O$ instead of lime, adjusting pH needed by an oxidation reaction, and the little lime only used as the carrier of successful settlement of indigo and indirubin. Step 3: Water refining The surfactant of protein or polypeptide in the suspension system of indigo, indirubin, and rough indigo are separated through nonspecific adsorption. Step 4: Substance change Ndole glycoside is transferred to indoxyl by enzymolysis, and indoxyl is formed to indole phenol-free radicals under aerobic conditions, one molecular indole phenol-free radical plus one molecule indole phenol to occur condensation to form one molecule leucoindigo, which then forms indigos under aerobic conditions; Once indoxyl is oxidized to isatin, one molecule isatin plus one molecule indole phenol to form indirubin. Step 5: Processing methods The indigos and indirubin could be directionality formed through studying the facts influencing the processing of Indigo Naturalis, which lays the foundation of normalization, controllability, and industrialization of processing of Indigo Naturalis.

实例二　基于传质、传热规律的传统的干馏蛋黄油炮制研究

研究对比了传统制备方法与现代超临界 CO_2 萃取方法进行蛋黄油的炮制，结果发现现代超临界萃取法卵磷脂提取物对烫伤动物模型治疗作用明确，为蛋黄油的制备提供了新的依据。研究采用 Box–Behnken 试验设计确定最佳工艺，并对其质量评价方面，进行了 β-谷甾醇薄层鉴别、相对密度、酸值、皂化值、碘值、过氧化值、水分与挥发物检查、微生物限度等在内的安全性及有效性研究，并以此为基础，起草了蛋黄油质量标准草案。

（引自江西中医药大学杨明主持的国家重点研发计划项目"10种传统特色炮制方法的传承、工艺技术创新与工业转化研究"；项目编号：2018YFC1707200）

实例三　鳖血柴胡炮制工艺与机制研究

基于中药炮制现代研究理论，以鳖血炒柴胡、鳖血润柴胡、酒柴胡、醋柴胡、生品柴胡为对象，利用 GC-MS、LC-MS、HPLC 等先进仪器与先进技术，开展柴胡南北成分鉴定、饮片炮制工艺、炮制品物质基础及退虚热作用的研究。研究构建了柴胡炮制物质基础变化及药理作用，柴胡炮制成分与入血成分、代谢成分与药理效应间的关系模型。

（引自江西中医药大学龚千锋主持的国家自然科学基金项目"樟帮特色鳖血柴胡炮制机制及品质研究"；项目编号：81260642）

Example 2 The Study on Processing of Traditional Distilled Egg Yolk Oil Based on the Rules of Mass Transfer and Heat Transfer

The traditional processing method and modern supercritical CO_2 extraction method to prepare egg yolk oil are compared, the results show that egg yolk oil processed by supercritical CO_2 extraction method has an exact therapeutic effect, which provides the new basis for the preparation of egg yolk oil with a new method. The optimum technology of egg yolk oil is also studied by Box-Behnken design, and the identification of TCL of β-rhamno, the determination of relative density, acid value, saponification value, iodine value, peroxide value, and the contents of water and volatiles, the microbial limit are as the contents of quality standards, basing on the index mentioned above, the draft of quality standards is formed.

Example 3 The Study on Processing Method and Mechanism of Bupleuri Radix Stir-fried with Turtle Blood

Based on the theories of processing, the Bupleuri Radix stir-fried with turtle blood, Bupleuri Radix soaked with turtle blood, Bupleuri Radix stir-fried with wine, Bupleuri Radix stir-fried with vinegar, and unprocessed Bupleuri Radix are compared. The GC-MS、LC-MS、and HPLC are applied to identify the difference between Bupleuri Scorzoneraefolii Radix and Bupleurum Radix, such as the processing technologies, the active substances and the effects of reducing fever due to deficiency of qi, etc. The models of active substances relating to pharmacological effects, the substances changed after processing relating to the blood composition, the metabolic composition relating to pharmacological effects are established.

实例四 基于药辅合一的药汁制法炮制研究

药汁制法始见于南朝刘宋·雷敩的《雷公炮炙论》，因其在解毒减毒、引药归经、纠正偏性、增强疗效、产生新作用、因病殊治扩大用药范围、精简处方等诸多方面具有显著意义，一直得以沿用。然而由于药汁制法操作烦琐，现代炮制品种越来越少，限制了临床使用和炮制方法传承。课题选取具有代表性的枳实制白术的药汁制饮片，应用现代药物化学、药理学方法对药辅合一的炮制工艺、炮制作用、质量标准进行详细研究，使药汁制法品种得到有效开发利用。建立了脾虚泄泻模型，考察不同配比枳实制白术饮片的"健脾祛燥"作用，筛选出枳实用量，再采用单因素试验和正交试验，以辛弗林及白术内酯Ⅲ含量为评价指标优选炮制工艺。研究发现其炮制作用与燥性主要成分苍术酮转化为具有健脾、抗癌活性的白术内酯Ⅰ、白术内酯Ⅲ有关，降低燥性同时提高其抗癌抑瘤、保肝健脾的功效。项目建立的分析方法系统适用性、重复性、准确性、稳定性良好。

（引自江西中医药大学杨明主持的国家重点研发计划项目"10种传统特色炮制方法的传承、工艺技术创新与工业转化研究"；项目编号：2018YFC1707200）

Example 4 The Study on Medicine Juice Process Based on Rules of Drugs plus Supplement

Medicine juice process method is the first record in *Lei's Treatise on Preparing Drugs* and still used up to now for the reasons of its pharmacological effects of detoxification and attenuation, inducing drug to meridian, moderating drugs' natures, enforcing the curative effect, producing new effects, expanding the indications for curative treatment, and simplifying prescription. But because the medicine juice process method is complicated, the samples used today become less and less, which limits the clinical use and inheritance of traditional processing methods. The pieces of Atractylodis Macrocephaly Rhizoma processed with the juice of Aurantii Fructus Immaturus are chosen to further study, the processing technology, processing effects, and quality standardization are studied to make further application of this kind pieces. The model of splenasthenic diarrhea is set to observe the difference of invigorating the spleen and removing dryness effect between the different ratios of Atractylodis macrocephaly rhizoma and the juice of Aurantii Fructus Immaturus. After screening the best ratio of Atractylodis macrocephaly rhizoma and the juice of Aurantii Fructus Immaturu, the contents of Synephrine and Atractylenolide III are used as the index to optimum processing technology. The results of the research also revealed that the processing effects are relative to the change of contents, after processing, atractylone is transferred to atractylode I and atractylode III with the effects of spleen-invigorating and anticancer. The processing effects include reducing dryness and anticancer, anti-tumor, protecting the liver, and strengthening the spleen either.

实例五　天南星科有毒中药矾制解毒的共性规律研究

天南星科 4 种有毒中药半夏、掌叶半夏、天南星、禹白附中具有共性的毒性物质主要是植物中含有的特殊针样晶体的毒针晶，该毒针晶由草酸钙、毒蛋白等组成。4 种有毒中药的毒针晶晶体细长尖锐、质地坚韧，表面带有倒刺和凹槽，中毒时可直接刺入机体组织，促发严重的炎症反应，毒针晶毒性（LD50）是相应生品的 200 倍以上。项目发现毒针晶的毒性与毒针晶针样晶体结构和毒针晶带有的毒蛋白相关。项目首次发现 4 种毒针晶带有的毒蛋白是相应植物中的凝集素蛋白。从 4 种有毒中药中分离纯化获得的 4 种凝集素蛋白和毒针晶均可诱导中性粒细胞迁移，显著诱导炎症因子释放，毒针晶及凝集素均可产生强烈促炎作用。毒针晶的毒性与毒针晶带有的毒蛋白"凝集素蛋白"的促炎作用相关。项目初步阐明天南星科 4 种有毒中药产生刺激性毒性的共性机制是"毒针晶直接刺入机体组织或细胞产生机械刺激，同时毒针晶上带有的凝集素蛋白随针晶的刺入进入机体组织，诱导中性粒细胞迁移、炎症因子大量释放、促发炎症反应；针晶独特晶型产生的机械刺激和凝集素蛋白诱发的促炎效应共同导致严重的炎症刺激性毒性"。项目研究表明，8% 白矾溶液炮制天南星科 4 种有毒中药的炮制解毒共性机制是"8% 白矾溶液中的 Al^{3+} 可与毒针晶草酸钙中的 $H_2C_2O_4$ 结合形成草酸铝络合物，使组成毒针晶的草酸钙溶解，毒针晶针样晶体结构破坏，产生机械刺激的物质基础被破坏；同时白矾溶液可以使毒针晶带有的凝集素蛋白水解、溶解或变性，凝集素蛋白的促炎作用下降，两者的共同作用导致 4 种有毒中药的刺激性毒性急剧降低"。

（引自南京中医药大学吴皓主持的国家自然科学基金项目"半夏刺激性毒性的物质基础及炮制解毒机理研究"；项目编号：30772785）

Example 5 The Study on Common Regulation of Detoxification of Toxic Chinese Medical Herbs in Araceaen Processed with Alummen

The four Chinese medical herbs of Pinelliae Rhizoma, Pinelliae Rhizoma Pedatisecta, Arisaematis Rhizoma, and Typhoni Rhizoma in Araceaen have the common toxic component which is called toxic needle-like calcium oxalate crystals, consisting of calcium oxalate, toxic protein, and so on. The needle-like calcium oxalate crystals in the four Chinese medical herbs are slender and sharp, hard texture, being with barb and fillister, which can stick into the body tissue, inducing serious inflammatory reactions. The LD50 value of needle-like calcium oxalate crystals is 200 times that of raw herbs. It is believed that the toxicity is relative to the structure and toxic protein of needle-like calcium oxalate crystals. Four kinds of toxic proteins are lectin protein existing in corresponding plants. This four lectin protein and toxic needle-like crystals could induce neutrophil migration, significantly induce inflammatory factor release, and have a strong proinflammatory effect. The proinflammatory effect of lectin protein is considered as relating to the toxicity of toxic needle-like crystals. The common mechanism of irritation toxicity of four toxic Chinese medical herbs is thought as, the needle-like crystals directly stick into the body tissue or cells to induce mechanical irritation, the lectin protein in the needle-like crystals then get into the body tissue as the sticking of needle-like crystals, inducing neutrophil migration, promoting the release of inflammatory factor, leading to an inflammatory reaction. The mechanical irritation produced by needle-like crystals and the proinflammatory effect induced by lectin protein lead to acute inflammatory and irritation toxicity together. The common mechanism of detoxification of four Chinese toxic herbs processed with 8% Alumen solution is, Al^{3+} in 8% Alumen solution could combine with $H_2C_2O_4$ in needle-like crystals to inform aluminum oxalate complex, make crystals in needle-like crystals resolve, the structure of needle-like crystals and the substance inducing mechanical irritation to be destroyed. At the same time, Alumen solution could hydrolyze, resolve or cause the lectin protein in needle-like crystals denaturation, reducing the proinflammatory effect of lectin protein. The common effects induce the irritation toxicity of the four Chinese medical herbs sharp decrease.

实例六　基于"析霜"特色的江西姜厚朴减毒增效炮制机制研究

项目运用星点设计-效应面法优选江西樟帮姜厚朴炮制工艺，确定最佳工艺参数。研究表明，樟帮姜厚朴炮制方法与《中国药典》所载姜厚朴存在较大差异，区别在于将厚朴与姜汁拌匀闷润至透，小火炒至药物表面黑褐色后，须晾凉后闷润至饮片出霜方可使用；课题还采用了化学成分和药效研究方法，从多方面对樟帮姜厚朴经特色炮制工艺炮制后，其成分与药效作用与药典法炮制姜厚朴的差异性进行研究，并采用主成分分析-人工神经网络（PCA-ANN）技术对厚朴各个炮制品种的指纹图谱与各项药效指标进行关联性分析，以各炮制品共有峰的相对峰面积行主成分分析，选取人工神经网络输入，以各项药效指标作为神经网络的输出，构建指纹图谱与各项药效指标之间的网络模型，阐明谱-效关系，揭示炮制机制。通过课题研究，得出结论认为：江西特色炮制工艺制得姜厚朴的"厚朴霜"为厚朴酚、和厚朴酚析出的混合物；江西樟帮姜霜厚朴不具备急性毒性和明显刺激性，在抗炎、镇痛、胃肠功能方面优于生品厚朴和《中国药典》姜厚朴，厚朴析霜对于厚朴的药效发挥具有积极意义；运用PCA技术筛选厚朴的主要有效成分，并使用人工神经网络关联厚朴指纹图谱中各个峰及各药效作用，分析得到在厚朴析霜后成分比例关系下，可使厚朴药效发挥到较佳水平。课题研究有利于提升传统中药炮制工艺技术，对具有鲜明地方特色的江西"樟帮"炮制技术研究奠定基础。

（引自江西中医药大学钟凌云主持的国家自然科学基金项目"基于'析霜'特色的江西姜厚朴减毒增效炮制机制研究"；项目编号：81060342）

第三部分　现代研究

Part III Modern Research of PCHM

Example 6 The Study on Processing Mechanism of Detoxification and Synergism of Magnoliae Officinalis Cortex Processed with Ginger Juice with Method Record in Zhangshu Branch in Jiangxi province Based on the Character of Frost Formation

The processing technology of Magnoliae Officinalis Cortex processed with ginger juice record in Zhangshu branch in Jiangxi province is optimized with central composite design-response surface methodology. The result shows that the processing technology of Magnoliae Officinalis Cortex in Zhangshu branch in Jiangxi province is different from that record in *Pharmacopoeia of the People's Republic of China*. As the method in Jiangxi province, the pieces of Magnoliae Officinalis Cortex are not only mixed and moistened with ginger juice and then stir-fried with low heat to drug surface in black-brown, but also the pieces should be cooled and moistened until the pieces are frosted before using. The composition and pharmacological effects are also compared to reveal the difference between Magnoliae Officinalis Cortex processed with method record in Zhangshu branch and Pharmacopoeia of the People's Republic of China separately. The PCA-ANN is applied to analyze the relationship between the fingerprint and pharmacological index of Magnoliae Officinalis Cortex processed with different methods. The common peaks in the fingerprint of different processing products are used to do principal component analysis, selecting artificial neural network as input, each pharmacological index as neural network output, network model of fingerprint and pharmacological index is set up, to clarify the spectrum-effect relationship and then the processing mechanism. It is believed that the frost secreted from Magnoliae Officinalis Cortex processed with ginger juice according to the method in Jiangxi province consists of magnolol and honokiol. Magnoliae Officinalis Cortex processed with Jiangxi method has no acute toxicity and apparent irritation. The effects of anti-inflammatory, analgesic and gastrointestinal functions of Magnoliae Officinalis Cortex processed with Jiangxi method are better than those of Magnoliae Officinalis Cortex processed with Pharmacopoeia of People's Republic of China method. The frost formation plays a positive role in the efficacy of Magnolia Officinalis. After the main active substances are screen with PCA, and the artificial neural network is associated with each peak and its pharmacological action in Magnoliae Officinalis Cortex, the conclusion is that under the condition of frost formation, the ratio of active substance get the best and could make better pharmacological effects of Magnoliae Officinalis Cortex. The research is beneficial to promote processing technology and lay a foundation for the research on processing technology of Jiangxi Zhangshu branch with distinct local characteristics.

实例七 "盐炙入肾－肾主骨"的物质基础和作用机制研究

选择"肾主骨"作用为切入点,研究盐制与咸入肾、肾主骨理论的相关性规律。采用成骨细胞模型,以增殖率为指标,筛选出续断、杜仲和牛膝三种药物的最佳炮制品即盐炙品的制备工艺,并以它们单味药及其药方、药对为实验载体,以促进骨生长、在与肾相关的组织和血液中的分布情况为指标,证明了盐炙后促进了它们入肾、主骨的作用;建立了各实验样品的化学数据库和活性数据库,采用多种数学分析法,凝练得到了以化学成分群动态变化和活性相关的数字化炮制品质量评价新模式,确定了各盐炙品药物化学成分群的合理波动范围,药物盐炙过程当中的盐热共同作用是药物增强入肾主骨作用的主要因素和机制。本课题采用了整体观策略进行研究,以实验数据揭示了中药盐炙与咸入肾、肾主骨理论的相关性及其机制,初步探索了炮制品质量优劣数字化评价新模式。

(引自成都中医药大学胡昌江主持的国家自然科学基金项目"基于益智仁盐炙前后及分别组成缩泉丸来研究'盐炙入肾－肾主水'的机制";项目编号:81473353)

Example 7 The Substances and Mechanism Study on 'Salt Roasting into Kidney-the Kidney Being in Charge of Bone'

The theory of "the kidney being in charge of bone" is the breakthrough point to study the relevant regulation of processing with saltwater and the theory of 'Salt Roasting into Kidney, the kidney being in charge of bone'. The Osteoblast model is applied in the research, the reproduction rate is an index to optimize the best processing technology of Dipsaci Radix, Eucommiae Cortex, and Achyranthis Bidentatae Radix processed with saltwater. The effect of promoting bone growth and distribution condition of drugs' composition in the renal-related tissue and blood is observed after administration of single drugs and their prescriptions. The results confirmed the theory 'Salt roasting into the kidney, the kidney being in charge of bone'. The chemistry databases and activity databases are set up in this research, many kinds of mathematical analysis methods are applied to establish a new model of digital processing quality evaluation about dynamic changes of chemical composition groups and activities. The reasonable fluctuation range of chemical composition is determined. The effect of heating together with salt is the main reason and mechanism of 'Salt Roasting into Kidney, the kidney being in charge of bone'. The research adopts a wholistic strategy to reveal the relationship between processing with salt and the theory of 'Salt Roasting into Kidney, the kidney being in charge of bone', establishing a new digital model to evaluate the quality of processed products.

实例八　基于栀子"炒炭存性"的科学内涵探究

　　课题开展栀子饮片的化学成分研究，从中分离鉴定了 20 个化学成分。比较研究了栀子饮片 2 个检测波长下 HPLC 指纹图谱特征，并结合主要色谱峰指认和 HPLC-MS/MS 分析，鉴定生栀子 13 个色谱峰、栀子炭 9 个色谱峰，初步阐释了栀子炒炭前后 HPLC 指纹图谱变化规律，基本明确了栀子不同饮片的化学成分组成。同时以 GC-MS 法首次对栀子炒炭前后低极性成分进行了比较分析，基本阐明了该类成分的变化趋势和成分组成。研究发现栀子炒炭后主要成分均大幅降低，但环烯醚萜类主成分组成变化不大，二萜色素成分组成发生变化显著。4 个主成分组合的模拟加热实验证明了二萜色类成分发生了苷类成分的降解、转化再到被破坏的过程，与 HPLC 指纹图谱和主成分定量分析研究结果一致。栀子鞣质类成分炭品较生品略有升高。亚甲蓝法吸附力测定结果显示栀子炭强于生栀子，栀子炒炭后仍具有抗炎和降温作用，证明栀子"炒炭存性"；栀子炒炭后能明显缩短 PT 时间，血栓长度增加，证实栀子炒炭后止血作用增强。

　　（引自中国中医科学院中药研究所张村主持的国家自然科学基金项目"基于栀子'炒炭存性'的科学内涵探究"；项目编号：30973943）

Example 8 The Scientific Connotation Study on 'Carbonizing by Stir-frying with Function Preserve' of Gareniae Fructus

The chemical compositions in Gareniae Fructus are analyzed and 20 compositions separated and identified. Comparing the characters of HPLC fingerprint under two detection wavelengths of slices of Gareniae Fructus, combining with the identification of main chromatographic peaks and HPLC-MS/MS analysis, 13 chromatographic peaks in raw Gareniae Fructus and 9 chromatographic peaks in carbonized Gareniae Fructus are identified. It preliminary reveals the change regulation of HPLC fingerprint of Gareniae Fructus before and after carbonizing, the compositions in Gareniae Fructus processed with different methods are determined either. At the same time, the low polar composition in Gareniae Fructus before and after carbonizing is compared by GC-MS. The changing trend and composition of the low polar composition are also basically determined. It is found that after carbonizing, the contents of the main composition in Gareniae Fructus decrease sharply, while the main constituents of iridoid terpenoids don't change much, and the composition of diterpenoid pigments changes significantly. A simulated heating test of combinations of four principal compositions ensures that the procedure of degradation, transformation, and destruction of diterpenoid pigments glycosides, which shows no difference from the results of HPLC fingerprint and quantitative analysis of major constituents. The contents of tannins are a little higher in carbonized Gareniae Fructus than those in raw Gareniae Fructus. Adsorptive power of carbonized Gareniae Fructus is stronger than that of raw Gareniae Fructus, and the carbonized Gareniae Fructus remains anti-inflammatory and hypothermic effects, which proves the theory 'carbonizing by stir-frying with function preserve'. Meanwhile, the PT time of carbonized Gareniae Fructus administration group is shorter than that of the raw carbonized Gareniae Fructus administration group, and the thrombus length also increases in carbonized Gareniae Fructus group, which affirms the hemostasis effect of carbonized Gareniae Fructus enhanced.

实例九　基于"寒热药性变化"的黄连炮制研究

基于"以热制寒"的典型炮制品种案例姜黄连，通过黄连姜制前后在药性表征和药效指标变化导向下的药性及药效物质基础变化研究，并将药性表征－药效－物质基础三者变化进行有机关联分析，深入系统阐明姜制黄连炮制机制。同时，结合多指标成分优化典型寒热药的"从制"与"反制"即黄酒制黄连和胆汁制黄连炮制工艺，研究结果与传统的"酒炙黄连以热制寒，缓和黄连苦寒之性；胆汁炙黄连使寒者益寒，增强黄连的苦寒之性"的炮制理论相一致。初步回答了炮制为何以及怎样影响寒热药性的问题，建立了"制法－药性"的现代炮制理论。

（引自江西中医药大学钟凌云主持的国家自然科学基金项目"基于药性表征－药效－物质基础关联的姜黄连炮制机理研究"；项目编号：81260643）

实例十　基于多种热力学形态水火共制熟三七炮制研究

通过考察三七炮制前后的药理药效作用特点，重点关注熟三七在补气和血、辅助抗肿瘤等方面的应用，研究结果表明熟三七具有补血、补气、辅助抗肿瘤的药理作用，并且在一定程度上反映了三七"生打熟补"的作用特点。用多指标成分正交设计法，优选最佳热力学形态三七炮制工艺，依据《饮片炮制规范研究指导原则》及相关技术规范，对熟三七性状、鉴别、检查、功能主治等项也进行研究，制定出完善的饮片质量标准。炮制方法和质量标准被《四川省中药饮片炮制规范》（2015年版）收载。

（引自江西中医药大学杨明主持的国家重点研发计划项目"10种传统特色炮制方法的传承、工艺技术创新与工业转化研究"；项目编号：2018YFC1707200）

Example 9 The Study on Processing of Goptidis Rhizoma Based on the Theory of 'Changes of Cold and Hot Properties'

The Goptidis Rhizoma processed with ginger juice is the typical example of 'Moderating drugs' cold nature by processing with hot nature supplement'. In this research, under the guide of changes of pharmacological characters and pharmacodynamic indicators, the changes of pharmaceutical properties and active substances are studied, and the changes of pharmacological characters, pharmacodynamic and active substances are correlated analyzed to clarify the processing mechanism of Goptidis Rhizoma processed with ginger juice. Meanwhile, the processing technologies of the Goptidis Rhizoma processed with wine, called ' inhibitory processing', and the Goptidis Rhizoma processed with bile, called 'adjuvant processing', are optimized combining with several preferred index. The results are in accordance with the theory of 'processing Goptidis Rhizoma with wine could moderate the herb's cold nature, processing Goptidis Rhizoma with bile could strength the herb's cold nature'. This research answers the question that why and how processing influence cold or hot properties of Chinese medical herbs, helping to build modern 'processing property theory,

Example 10 The Study on Processed Notoginseng Radix Et Rhizoma Based on Hydrothermal Copolymerization of Various Thermodynamic Forms

The pharmacological effects of Notoginseng Radix Et Rhizoma before and after processing, especially the effects of supplementing qi and blood, assisting anti-Tumor, are observed. The results show that processed Notoginseng Radix Et Rhizoma does have the effects of supplementing qi and blood and assisting anti-Tumor, which reflects the characteristics of Notoginseng Radix Et Rhizoma's function of "raw product beating, processed product tonifying" to a certain extent. A multi-index orthogonal experimental design is applied to optimize the best thermodynamic form processing technology. On another side, according to the *Guiding Principles for Research on Processing Standards of Chinese Herbal Pieces* and other relative technical specifications, the characters, identification, examination, functional indications of processed Notoginseng Radix Et Rhizoma are also studied to establish a perfect quality standard for decoction pieces. The processing technology and quality standard are all collected in *Processing Specification of Traditional Chinese Medicine Pieces in Sichuan Province* (2015 Edition)

实例十一 江西特色蜜麸枳壳减燥增效炮制机制研究

通过优选蜜麸枳壳炮制工艺，并基于枳壳燥性损伤机体津液的科学假说，拟通过对枳壳生、制品对健康大鼠肾 AQP3、血清 cAMP、血清 cGMP 含量的研究，比较不同炮制品燥性；并观察其对胃窦、结肠 c-kit、SCF 的 mRNA 表达的影响，在分子水平阐明枳壳蜜麸制"减燥"机制。此外，通过检测枳壳生、制品对功能性消化不良大鼠血清 VIP、CGRP、MTL 含量的影响，采用 Western Blot 与 IHC 法检测 GAS、SOM 蛋白在大鼠下丘脑和胃体的表达，阐明基于增强"行气宽中"作用的蜜麸枳壳"增效"炮制机制。

（引自江西中医药大学祝婧主持的国家自然科学基金项目"基于质量标志物在'炮制－药物代谢－生物效应'环节的变化关联探讨樟帮蜜麸枳壳炮制机理"；项目编号：82060716）

实例十二 传统炆制黄精的现代研究

结合多指标成分对建昌帮炆制黄精的炮制工艺进行筛选与优化，并对炆黄精及酒黄精、九蒸九晒黄精及黄精生品在炮制前后化学成分和药理作用进行系统研究。探讨不同火力和炮制状态下多糖水解而成的单糖与游离氨基酸发生美拉德反应，生成 5-羟甲基糠醛的变化情况，并结合抗疲劳、抗氧化、增强免疫动物实验发现，炆黄精药效作用机制可能与增加肝糖原储备、延长负重游泳力竭时间，调节 SOD、MDA 水平，并在一定程度上增强脾和胸腺的免疫功能有关。

（引自中国中医科学院中医基础理论研究所王淳主持的国家自然科学基金项目"免疫活性多糖级分导向的黄精与酒黄精质量评价方法研究"；项目编号：81603294）

Example 11 The Study on Processing Mechanism of Reduce Dryness and Increase Efficiency of Honey-Bran Stir-fried Auranii Fructus with Jiangxi Processing Character

The processing technology of honey-bran stir-fried Auranii Fructus is optimized. And then, based on the theory of 'dryness damages body fluid', the raw and processed Auranii Fructus are compared in the dryness through determining the contents of AQP3 in rats' kidney, cAMP, and cGMP in rats' serum, and observing the effect on mRNA level in c-kit, SCF of sinuses ventriculi and large intestine. The purpose is to clarify the mechanism of reducing drying of honey-bran stir-fried Auranii Fructus at the molecular level. Meanwhile, the contents of VIP、CGRP、MTL in serum of rats with functional dyspepsia are determined in raw and processed Auranii Fructus, and the level of proteins of GAS and SOM in rats' thalamus and gastric are also observed with western blot and IHC. The purpose is to clarify the processing mechanism of increasing efficiency of promoting qi circulation to alleviate the middle energizer of honey-bran stir-fried Auranii Fructus.

Example 12 The Modern Study on Processing of Traditional Simmering Polygonati Rhizoma

The processing technology of simmering Polygonati Rhizoma is optimized by combining the contents of several compositions, and the composition and pharmacological effects of simmering Polygonati Rhizoma, wine stir-fried Polygonati Rhizoma, multiple steaming and sunning Polygonati Rhizoma, and raw Polygonati Rhizoma. The Maillard reaction occurred by the monosaccharide hydrolyzed from polysaccharide and free amino acid under different heating power and processing is discussed, the change of product of 5-hydroxymethylfurfural is observed, combining with the experimental findings in effecting of resisting fatigue, antioxidant and enhancing immunity. The results show that the mechanism of the effect of simmering Polygonati Rhizoma may relate to increasing hepatic glycogen reserve, extending exhaustion time of weight-bearing swimming, regulating of SOD and MDA levels, and increasing the immunologic function of spleen and thymus to some degree.

实例十三 基于多物料、多流程的传统炮附子炮制研究

在传承创新濒临失传的附子传统"炮法"基础上，首创微波炮附子关键技术，通过化学、药理与毒效关系研究，证明微波炮附子毒性最小，具有特殊免疫促进与抗心肌缺血功能，并将专利技术实现产业化应用。同时，首次揭示乌头碱与甘草酸相互作用难溶性沉淀的减毒机制，证实"附子得甘草则缓"的科学内涵，奠定了甘草炮制减毒的原创思维；芍药苷抑制乌头碱的肠吸收以降低在心、肝、肾脏器的蓄积毒性，诠释白芍与附子配伍减毒的科学性。同时以精准的毒效评价攸关临床用药的安全优效。采用UPLC-MS-Q-TOF结合植物代谢组学方法，从附子中鉴定生物碱50余种，研究确定道地优质附子的质量标志物。首次建立毒性与含量整合的毒性成分指数，实现成分对毒性的精准预测；基于急性心衰模型与谱效关联，证明去甲猪毛菜碱是附子强心的关键质量标志物。以此为基础，系统阐明叶型、产地、规格、浸胆、炮制对附子毒效与优质性的影响规律；首创鲜附子定尺切丁、一步减毒、当量一致的新型精标饮片，大幅简化炮制工艺，实现提质增效、绿色制造，且强心、温阳活性显著强于传统饮片。

（引自江西中医药大学杨明主持的国家重点研发计划项目"10种传统特色炮制方法的传承、工艺技术创新与工业转化研究"；项目编号：2018YFC1707200）

Part III Modern Research of PCHM

Example 13 The Study on Traditional Blast-fried Aconiti Lateralis Radix Praeparata Based on Multiple Supplements and Steps

The processing technology of blast-fried Aconiti Lateralis Radix Praeparata with microwave is first found based on traditional technology of stir-frying of Aconiti Lateralis Radix Praeparata. Through the study on the relationship between composition, pharmacology, and toxic effect, it is proved that the toxicity of blast-fried Aconiti Lateralis Radix Praeparata with microwave is the least compared to other processed Aconiti Lateralis Radix Praeparata. At the same time, these processed products also have the effects of special immune promotion and anti-myocardial ischemia. 50 kinds of alkaloids are identified through UPLC-MSQ-TOF and metabonomics, quality markers of high-quality genuine Aconiti Lateralis Radix Praeparata are determined. Toxicity-component index about toxicity and composition contents is first found to realize accurate prediction of the relationship between composition and toxicity. The salsolinol is approved as the key quality marker with cardiotonic effect in Aconiti Lateralis Radix Praeparata based on the relationship between acute heart failure model and spectral effect. On this basis, the regulation of toxicity and high quality of Aconiti Lateralis Radix Praeparata influenced by leaf shape, origination, specification, bile impregnated, and processing is discovered. A new type of refined and standard slices of fresh Aconiti Lateralis Radix Praeparata with cutting lump, one step detoxification, and the identical equivalent weight is firstly initiated, which simplify the processing technology, realize the quality and efficiency improvement, and green manufacturing, the new type slices show better effects of cardiotonic and warming yang than traditionally processed slices.

实例十四 基于 UHP-MS/MS 和化学分析法对天麻炮制品中的主成分分析

天麻是中国传统医学史上最早也是最重要的预防和治疗神经性和神经性疾病的中草药之一。它所含的生物活性成分，具有明显的潜在医疗价值，并已开展了研究。然而，天麻在临床使用前，必须进行炮制。

天麻经过炮制后，其成分含量、成分性质或者两者均有可能发生变化，进而影响到临床疗效。其炮制方法多样，如酒、蜂蜜、蒺藜、麦麸、浆液等，而"建昌帮"采用的炮制方法，则是将清蒸、切片后的天麻，与生姜汁混合，然后于室温下进行烘干即可。

尽管姜制天麻炮制品，在临床应用中具有较好的疗效，由于缺乏相应的科学资料，致使其临床应用受限。因此，弄清"建昌帮"姜制天麻炮制前后成分变化差异，是揭示炮制机制的关键，为临床应用提供依据。本研究建立了一种与主成分分析相结合的 UHPLC-MS/MS 分析方法，对天麻原材料、干燥品和姜制 5 天后的天麻样品进行了分析。

通过 MarkerLynx 软件，对 TOF-MS/MS 等化学方法获得的数据进行了多元统计分析，鉴定出了原药材、干燥品和姜制五天后等不同样品之间主成分差异。本研究结果表明，"建昌帮"炮制法能影响天麻主成分含量，说明该研究结果，将有助于揭示姜制天麻炮制机制和指导其临床应用。

（引自江西中医药大学叶喜德主持的国家自然科学基金项目"基于'姜制温散'理论的建昌帮天麻炮制的'药性 – 药效 – 效应成分'关联的炮制作用变化机理研究"；项目编号：81760712）

Example 14 Identification and Characterization of Key Chemical Constituents in Processed Gastrodiae Rhizoma Using UHPLC-MS/MS and Chemometric Methods

Gastrodiae Rhizoma is one of the earliest and most important traditional Chinese herbal medicine for the prevention and treatment of neuralgic and nervous diseases for centuries in the history of traditional Chinese medicine (TCM). Gastrodiae Rhizoma contains bioactive compounds, which have been come to highlight some of their potential therapeutic values and have developed the subject of extensive research. However, Gastrodiae Rhizoma has to be processed before clinical application.

The processed Gastrodiae Rhizoma can raise the change of these ingredients in content, potentially in chemical property or both of them, and influence its clinical efficacy. There are many processing ways including Gastrodiae Rhizoma mixed with wine, honey, Tribulus Terrestris, wheat bran, or serofluid, but the "Jianchang Society" processing method is to mix steamed and sliced Gastrodiae Rhizoma with ginger juice, then dried at room temperature.

Although the processed product of Gastrodiae Rhizoma with ginger has practically shown good efficacy, there is a limitation for its clinical application owing to the lack of scientific evidence. Therefore, finding out the difference of chemical composition in Gastrodiae Rhizoma proposed by the "Jiangchang Society" method before and after processing is the key to reveal the concoction mechanism for providing clinical application. In this study, a UHPLC-MS/MS associated with principal component analysis has been developed for the analysis of Gastrodiae Rhizoma raw material, dried Gastrodiae Rhizoma, and samples that Gastrodiae Rhizoma processed with ginger juice and dried for 5 days (GEP5D).

The primary marker compounds diversifications between different grouping samples such as raw vs dried and raw vs GEP5D are determined after the TOF MS and MS/MS data are applied for multivariate statistical analysis using MarkerLynx software. This result inferred that the processing way of Gastrodiae Rhizoma by the "Jiangchang" Society method affected the contents of Gastrodiae Rhizoma's principal composition and is helpful to understand the processing mechanism and clinical application in traditional Chinese medicine.

实例十五　药代/毒代动力学技术在中药炮制现代研究中的应用

药代/毒代动力学技术能够有效地发现经过中药炮制之后药物在体内的吸收、分布、代谢、排泄和毒性改变的情况（ADME/T），能科学地阐明传统中药炮制的科学内涵。研究运用了药代/毒代动力学技术研究草乌与生半夏、法半夏配伍毒代动力学变化，设给药前和给药后共13个采血时间点，采用LC-MS/MS检测血浆样品中主要毒性成分草乌中双酯型生物碱的含量，血药浓度-时间数据经DAS2.0软件处理计算毒代动力学参数。结果发现，草乌与生半夏、法半夏配伍，3个毒性成分的AUC（0-t）有显著区别，说明炮制影响了毒性成分的吸收程度，乌头碱与新乌头碱含量在草乌与法半夏配伍后明显降低，与生半夏配伍后明显增大；草乌与生半夏、法半夏配伍，3个毒性成分的Cmax有显著区别，说明炮制改变了毒性成分的吸收速率，新乌头碱和次乌头碱含量，醇提草乌与法半夏配伍后降低，结论认为，草乌与生半夏配伍，双酯型生物碱（主要的毒性成分）的吸收程度与速率增加，草乌与法半夏配伍后，双酯型生物碱的吸收程度与速率减小，草乌与法半夏配伍降低了毒性。

（引自南京中医药大学吴皓主持的国家自然科学基金项目"基于炎症级联反应的天南星科有毒中药毒性作用机制和生姜解毒机理研究"；项目编号：81573605）

Example 15 The Application of Pharmacokinetics and Toxicokinetics in Modern Research of Chinese Medicine Herbs Processing

The changes in absorption, distribution, metabolism, excretion, and toxicity in vivo (ADME/T) of drugs can be discovered through pharmacokinetics and toxicokinetics, and then the scientific connotation of traditional processing could be exactly expressed through these techniques. The change of toxicokinetics of compatibility of Aconiti Kusnezoffii Radix and Pinelliae Rhizoma or Pinellinae Rhizoma Praeparatum is studied with pharmacokinetics and toxicokinetics, 13-time points for blood collection are designed before and after administration, LC-MS/MS is applied to determine the main toxic composition of diester alkaloids in samples serum, the parameter of toxicokinetics is calculated through DAS2.0 based on the blood concentration-time data.

The results show that, after compatibility of Aconiti Kusnezoffii Radix and Pinelliae Rhizoma or Pinellinae Rhizoma Praeparatum, the AUC (0-t) of three toxic compositions shows a significant difference, which explains that processing influences the absorption degree of toxic composition. The contents of aconitine and neoaconitine decrease after compatibility of Aconiti Kusnezoffii Radix and Pinellinae Rhizoma Praeparatum, but increase after compatibility of Aconiti Kusnezoffii Radix and Pinelliae Rhizoma. The Cmax shows a significant difference between three toxic compositions after compatibility of Aconiti Kusnezoffii Radix and Pinelliae Rhizoma or Pinellinae Rhizoma Praeparatum, which explains that processing change the absorption rate of the toxic composition. The contents of neoaconitine and hypaaconitine are also decreased after compatibility of Aconiti Kusnezoffii Radix and Pinellinae Rhizoma Praeparatum. The conclusion is that the absorption degree and rate of toxic composition increase after compatibility of Aconiti Kusnezoffii Radix and Rhizoma Pinelliae Rhizomae , but decrease after compatibility of Aconiti Kusnezoffii Radix and Pinellinae Rhizoma Praeparatum. The compatibility of Aconiti Kusnezoffii Radix and Pinellinae Rhizoma Praeparatum could decrease the toxicity.

第九章　现代炮制研究展望

中药炮制是我国人民经过数千年的医疗实践，不断总结、改进、发展而形成的传统制药技术。中药材经过炮制后直接应用于临床或供中成药生产用的药物即"中药饮片"，是中医用药的物质基础，但中药饮片因多种化学成分共存，作用有多方向、多靶点的特点，"炮制不明，药性不确"，应用要遵循"生熟异用、生熟有度"的原则，因此，采用合适的炮制工艺、保障中药饮片的质量是深入探讨炮制工艺、确保中药临床用药安全、有效的关键。

迄今为止，中药炮制的发展历经了几千年的历史，炮制技术从原始的手工化生产到作坊式生产再到机械化生产，炮制标准从最初的经验性状鉴别到内在成分的检测，炮制理论从单纯的炮制前后功效对比到更深入的科学内涵研究，都揭示了中药炮制学这门古老的学科在与时俱进，并取得了巨大的发展。但是，由于中药材及中药饮片的来源、加工及应用上的特殊性，中药炮制的发展依然受到了一定的限制，在很多方面须改进和完善。

Part III Modern Research of PCHM

Chapter Nine   Research Outlook of PCHM

PCHM is related to the traditional pharmaceutical technology which has been summed up, improved, and developed by the Chinese people after thousands of years of medicinal practice. After being processed, CMM (Chinese Materia Medica) can be directly used in the clinic or made into herbal slices which are the materials for the production of Chinese patent drugs. It is the material basis of TCM. However, due to the coexistence of many chemical compositions, the action of CMM has the characteristics of multi-direction and multi-targets. "The processing method is unknown and the medicinal property is not definite", so the application of processing methods should be based on the principle of " different usage of raw and processed materials, and proper processing methods of raw and processed materials". Therefore, adopting proper processing technology and ensuring the quality of traditional Chinese medicine pieces is the key to discuss the processing technology and ensure the safety and effectiveness of traditional Chinese medicine.

Up to now, PCHM has developed thousands of years, and processing technology has developed from original manual production to workshop production and mechanized production. Meanwhile, processing standards have been from the initial empirical identification to the detection of internal composition. The processing theory has changed from the simple comparison of the efficacy before and after processing to the more scientific in-depth study. All of those reveals that the ancient discipline of PCHM is keeping pace with the times and has made great achievements. But due to the source of CMM and herbal slices, and the particularity of processing and application, the development of PCHM is still limited and improvements should be done in many aspects.

一、药材产地初加工、饮片炮制真正做到工艺规范化、规模化、产业化和一体化

中药饮片产业是传统中药三大支柱产业之一，中药饮片质量的好坏直接关系着临床疗效是否能准确、充分地发挥。如何保证中药饮片的质量，除了药材来源，产地初加工、饮片炮制工艺稳定是最重要的影响因素。

1. 产地初加工

产地药材加工是形成商品药材前处理的加工过程，是药材品质、性状特征与质量形成的重要环节。中药大部分来源于植物，产地初加工主要包括采收后的净制、干燥、切制处理等。其中净制中及切制前的水处理环节及药材或饮片的干燥环节尤为重要。近年来，广大医药工作者在中药材产地加工相关方面进行了大量的研究和改进，但由于药材产地不同、品质不同及各地传统加工习惯不同等诸多因素，相同药材产地初加工的工艺多有不同，导致药材质量良莠不齐，很多药材及饮片依然缺乏统一的质量判定标准，给市场监管部门带来了困扰的同时，也使饮片市场较为混乱。例如，白芍道地产区加工方法有煮后去皮和去皮后煮两种，有研究显示，两种加工方法加工出的药材外观和有效成分的含量存在很大差异，而且是色泽较差的加工品有效成分的含量很高。另有研究显示，附子产地加工过程中，对成分含量影响最大的环节是热处理蒸或煮，水处理、浸泡、漂对含量影响不大，故加热方式和时间应作为重要指标进行量化。在干燥方面，由于大型烘干机成本高，难以被广大农户接受，大多数农户采用硫黄浸泡烘干或硫黄燃烧密闭烘烤，易造成二氧化硫残留量超标而危害人们身体健康。

Part III Modern Research of PCHM

Section One   Roughly Processed CMM and the Processing of Herbal Slices Should be Truly Standardized, Scaled, Industrialized and Integrated.

The herbal slices industry is one of the three pillar industries of traditional Chinese medicines. The quality of herbal slices is directly related to whether the clinical efficacy is accurate and adequate. The rough processing and the stability of the processing technology of herbal slices as well as the sources of CMM are the most important factors in ensuring the quality of herbal slices.

1. Rough processing in the place of origin

The processing of CMM in their places of origin is the pre-processing of commercial medicinal materials, which is an important link of forming its fabric, characteristic, and quality of CMM. Most of the CMM are from plants and the primary processing mainly includes cleansing, drying, and cutting after collecting, etc. In the process of purification and cutting, water processing and drying of CMM or herbal slices are particularly important. In recent years, pharmaceutical workers have made much research and improvements in the primary processing of Chinese medicinal materials. However, different places of origin, quality, way of processing techniques, and rough processing of the same CMM result in uneven qualities. There is still a lack of unified quality standards in CMM and herbal pieces, which not only brings trouble to the market regulatory departments but also makes the market more chaotic. For example, there are two processing methods in the place of origin of Paeoniae Radix Alba (Baishao), that is, peeling after boiling and boiling after peeling. Studies have shown that the appearance of Paeoniae Radix Alba and the content of active composition produced by the two processing methods are very different, and the content of the active composition of the processed products with poor color is higher. Other studies have shown that in the primary processing of Aconiti Lateralis Radix Praeparata (Fuzi), the most important procedure affecting the content of composition is heat processing such as steaming, boiling, while water processing, soaking, and bleaching has little effect on the composition. So the heating mode and time should be quantified as an important index. In terms of drying, it is difficult for farmers to use some large-scale dryers because of their high cost. Most farmers dry medicines after sulfur soaking or burn sulfur to bake medicines in closed space, which is likely to cause excessive sulfur dioxide residue and endangers people's health.

鉴于此类现象，首先，医药工作者对产品初加工的环节应给予更大的重视，进一步加强对传统加工方法的传承与现代科学技术的结合，优化炮制工艺，制定切实可行的检测标准。中药炮制技术有几千年的历史，古人在医疗实践中在炮制方面总结了很多宝贵的经验。在《中医药创新发展规划纲要（2006—2020年）》中，国家明确将"开展中药饮片传统经验继承"放在优先领域；国家发改委颁布的《产业结构调整指导目录（2011）》中，将"中药饮片创新技术及运用"列为鼓励发展项目。为了力求继承与发展相结合，可以对传统炮制工艺深入研究，进行大数据统计处理，并借助现代的科技手段去验证并改进传统工艺，最大限度地保证药材的质量。

2. 产地初加工饮片炮制的一体化

中药材因产地、品质的差异，以及各地区习惯的不同等，同级别同药材的炮制方法亦常有很大不同，势必导致中药饮片的质量良莠不齐，直接影响临床疗效的发挥。而中药饮片的应用因多组分作用的特殊性，《中国药典》及各级炮制规范目前尚无法对中药材炮制的工艺描述给出量化指标，并且炮制一线的技术人员严重缺乏，也是造成目前饮片市场产生炮制乱象的原因之一。炮制工作者应在努力传承与发展的基础上，推进产地初加工和饮片炮制一体化，不仅可以有效减少不适当水处理和干燥的环节对药材及饮片质量的影响，并可同样大大降低"作坊式"生产因随机性造成的饮片质量上的差异，在保障中药材及饮片质量及加工规范化、规模化、产业化方面具有诸多优势，亦更容易实现将中药材生产的 GAP 要求与饮片生产的 GMP 要求相结合，力求从源头开始的每个环节做到中药材及饮片的质量达到稳定、可控。

Because of such phenomena, it is believed that, first of all, medical workers should pay more attention to the rough processing of products, and further strengthen the integration of traditional processing methods with modern science and technology, optimize the processing technology, and develop practical testing standards. PCHM technology has a history of thousands of years and the ancients summed up a lot of valuable experience in the field of processing in medical practice. For the combination of inheritance and development, in the outline of *Innovation and Development Plan of TCM (2006-2020)*, the government explicitly regulates that carrying out the heritage of traditional experience of herbal slices is prioritized; and in *the Guiding Catalogue of Industrial Structure Adjustment (2011)* promulgated by the National Development and Reform Commission, "innovative technology and application of herbal slices preparation" is listed as an incentive development project. For striving for a combination of inheritance and development, it is believed that the traditional processing technology can be studied deeply and that the traditional technology should be verified and improved by big data statistical processing and by the means of modern science and technology to maximize the high quality of CMM.

2. The Integration of the rough processing in places of origin and the processing of raw pieces

Due to the difference in origin and quality of CMM, as well as the different habits of different regions, the processing methods of the same grade and the same medicinal materials are often very different, which will inevitably lead to the uneven quality of Chinese herbal slices, which directly affects the clinical effect. However, because of the particularity of multicomponent reactions of Chinese herbal slices, the quantitative index for the description of the processing technics has not been stipulated by the *Chinese Pharmacopoeia* and the processing standards at all levels. At the same time, the lack of first-line processing technicians is also one of the reasons for the current chaos in the herbal slices market. Based on the efforts to inherit and develop, the processing workers should promote the integration of the rough processing in the production areas and the processing of herbal slices, which can not only effectively reduce the influence of inappropriate watering and drying processing on the quality of CMM and herbal slices, but also greatly reduce the difference in the quality of herbal slices randomly produced by workshop. It has many advantages in ensuring the quality of CMM and herbal slices and standardizing scale, and industrialized processing. It is also easier to combine the GAP requirements for the production of CMM with the GMP requirements for the production of herbal slices, and strives to achieve a stable and controllable quality of CMM and herbal slices at every stage from the source.

二、充分利用现代先进科技手段，真正做到传承与发展有机结合，进一步推进质量控制标准化、统一化

中药炮制的发展迄今已有几千年历史，传统的中药饮片质控方法大多是采用饮片的外观性状指标，如形、色、气、味、质等，通过眼看、手摸、鼻闻、口尝等方式来控制炮制品的质量，具有不可避免的主观性差异，缺乏严谨性，无法保障饮片质量的准确性和一致性。近年来，广大科技工作者通过努力，在饮片质控方面取得了一定的成绩，但由于中药多成分联合作用的复杂性、标准物质及对照药材、标准饮片难以获得等原因，中药饮片炮制的质量控制依然任重道远，须结合现代多种先进科技手段检测，大胆尝试，以药效学指标为标准，综合评价。

1. 在多成分定量、指纹图谱定性的基础上，结合药效学实验和生物效价测定，进一步完善质控评价机制

中药因其多成分、多靶点的临床特征，作用机制复杂，故中药饮片的质量评价一直是重点和难点问题。目前，传统经验鉴别与"多成分定量、指纹图谱定性"的现代科学方法相结合的饮片质量评价模式虽已建立，但因很多中药的有效成分归属、指标成分含量是否与临床疗效呈绝对正相关、不同有效成分单体生物效价如何等诸多实际问题尚未明确，中药材及饮片的质量评价依然存在很多缺陷。建议经验鉴别与"多成分定量、指纹图谱定性"结合为前提，将所选成分的生物效价测定纳入评价体系，结合药效学结果，多指标综合评定，使质控标准更科学、更完善。

Part III Modern Research of PCHM

Section Two Make Full Use of Modern Advanced Scientific Technology to Achieve the True Combination of Inheritance and Development, and Further Promote the Standardization and Unification of Quality Control

The development of PCHM has a history of thousands of years, and most of the traditional quality control methods have been adopted to judge and control the quality of processed products according to the appearance index of Chinese slices, such as the shape, color, smell, taste, texture, and so on, and by seeing with the eyes, touching with hands, smelling with noses and tasting with mouths, which inevitably differs in subjectivity and lacks rigorousness, so it is unable to ensure the accuracy and consistency of the quality of herbal slices. In recent years, a vast number of scientific and technological researchers have made certain achievements in the quality control of herbal slices through efforts. But due to the complexity of the multi-component combination of herbal slices, the difficulty to get reference materials, the control medicines and the standard pieces of CMM, and some other reasons, there is still a long way to go to control the quality of traditional Chinese medicine pieces, so it is necessary to test and try boldly with the modern advanced scientific and technological means, take the pharmacodynamics index as the standard, and evaluate comprehensively.

1. Based on multi-component quantification and fingerprint characterization, combining with pharmacodynamic experiments and bioavailability to further improve. the quality control evaluation mechanism

Because of its clinical characteristics of multi-component and multi-target, the mechanism of action of Chinese herbal medicine is complex. The quality evaluation of herbal slices has always been a key and difficult issue. At present, the quality evaluation model of the traditional experience identification methods combined with the modern scientific method of "multi-component quantitative, fingerprint characterization" has been established. However, many practical problems have not been solved, such as the uncertain effective composition of many TCM, whether the content of index composition is positively correlated with clinical efficacy, and what the bioavailability of monomers of different active compositions is. There are still many defects in the quality evaluation of CMM and herbal slices. It is suggested that the experience identification methods combined with the "multi-component quantitative and fingerprint mapping qualitative" as the premise, the bioavailability determination of the selected components should be included in the evaluation system, combined with the pharmacodynamics results and comprehensive evaluation of multiple indicators, so that the quality control standards are more scientific and perfect.

2. 传统经验结合新兴科技手段，综合应用

传统的经验鉴别依靠人的感官，存在着不可避免的主观性和随机性，故可考虑引入现代先进的科技成果，如电子鼻和电子舌、机器视觉技术等应用于饮片鉴别。

电子鼻采用了人工智能技术，实现了通过仪器"嗅觉"对产品进行的客观分析。由于这种智能传感器矩阵系统中配有不同类型传感器，能更充分更灵敏地模拟人类鼻子的功能，通过它可以得到该产品独特的信息，从而进行系统化与科学化的气味监测、鉴别、判断和分析。电子舌是根据模拟味觉感受机制来设计的，当味觉物质在薄膜上被吸收，数据便通过类脂膜上电位的变化而获得。然后由计算机对数据进行模式识别，得到反映样品味觉特征的结果。在炮制研究中，可用电子鼻和电子舌模拟人类感官来检测炮制品的气和味，并进行大数据对比分析、总结，或可作为饮片炮制标准的参考条件之一。

机器视觉技术，是通过多学科技术，用计算机来模拟、实现人的视觉功能，目前已广泛应用到国内外多个行业，其中红外光谱技术应用尤为广泛，近红外光谱在定量分析中多用，而中红外则在结构分析中占重要地位。中药饮片炮制前后及炮制过程中，饮片会发生复杂的理化变化，根据机器视觉技术捕捉到的信息变化，通过大数据分析，亦可用于中药炮制质控检测。目前，机器视觉技术不仅在无损鉴别药材的真伪和分级中有较大贡献，并已在中药炮制领域中开始应用且效果较好。

2. Comprehensive applications of traditional experience in combination with emerging scientific and technological means

Traditional experience identification relies on human senses, which means there is inevitable subjectivity and randomness. Therefore, the introduction of modern advanced scientific and technological achievements, such as electronic nose and tongue, machine vision technology for the identification of pieces can be considered.

The electronic nose adopts artificial intelligence technology to achieve an objective analysis of the product by smelling instruments. Because this intelligent sensing system is equipped with different types of sensors, it can more fully and sensitively simulate the function of the human nose, through which the unique information of the product can be obtained, thus, it can systematically and scientifically monitor, identify, judge and analyze odors. The electronic tongue is designed by simulating the taste sensation of humans. When the tasteful substance is absorbed on the film, the data is obtained by change of potential on the lipid-like membrane. The pattern recognition of the data is then obtained by the computer to get the result reflecting the taste characteristics of the sample. In the research of processing, electronic nose and electronic tongue simulate the human senses to detect the smell and taste of the processed products, then compares and summarizes the big data, which may be used as one of the reference conditions for the standard of herbal slices.

Machine vision technology is a multi-disciplinary technology that uses computers to simulate and realize human visual functions, which has been widely used in many industries at home and abroad. Among them, infrared spectroscopy is especially widely used. Near-infrared spectroscopy is usually used in quantitative analysis, while mid-infrared plays an important role in structural analysis. Before and after the processing of traditional Chinese medicine pieces, there will be complex physical and chemical changes. According to the change of information captured by machine vision technology, through big data analysis, it can also be used for quality control detection of traditional Chinese medicine processing. At present, machine vision technology not only contributes greatly to the non-destructive identification and classification of medicinal materials, but also has been applied in the field of PCHM research, and the effect is good.

3. 大数据分析、总结，多渠道检测，制定多指标综合评价模式，改进并完善质控标准

中医药独特的科学体系决定了中医用药的独特性，中药炮制是中医用药的特色，而多成分联合、多靶点作用，导致了中药材及饮片的质控标准难以制定，单纯以有效成分含量作为质控标准，会失去中医用药的特色和科学性，应在保持中药特殊性的基础上，将传统的判断标准与现代科技手段相结合，充分利用大数据分析、对比、总结、验证，改进并完善中药炮制的质控标准。

中药炮制是中医用药的特点，中药炮制直接关系着中药的临床疗效。在健全质控标准的基础上，改进炮制工艺，不仅有利于进一步探讨炮制理论，更能保证中药药效发挥的准确性与高效性。在科技发达的当代，炮制工作者应在继承炮制传统的基础上，集思广益，融合现代先进科学技术和思想，为中药炮制的发展及中医药现代化而努力。

3. Analysis and summary with big data, test through multi-channel, formulate a comprehensive evaluation model with multiple indicators to improve and make perfect quality control standards perfect

The unique scientific system of TCM determines the uniqueness of TCM. PCHM is a characteristic of TCM. The combination of multi-composition and multi-targets has made it difficult to formulate quality control standards for CMM and Chinese herbal medicine. Simply taking the content of some effective composition as the standard of quality control will lose the characteristics and scientific nature of TCM, so the traditional evaluation criteria should be combined with modern scientific and technological means based on maintaining the peculiarity of CMM, to improve and make the quality control standards of Chinese medicine processing refined through the analysis, comparison, summary and verification with big data.

PCHM is the feature of TCM, and it is directly related to the clinical efficacy of TCM. Improving the processing technology will not only help to further explore the processing theory but also ensure the accuracy and efficiency of Chinese medicine efficacy based on optimizing quality control standards. In the modern age of advanced science and technology, processing researchers should integrate modern science, technology, and ideas based on inheriting the processing tradition and benefit by mutual discussion, to make great efforts for the development of traditional Chinese medicine processing and the modernization of traditional Chinese medicine.

参考文献：

[1] 裴科，宁燕，蔡皓，等.基于HPLC指纹图谱结合化学模式识别的川芎炮制前后对比研究[J].中草药，2021，52（05）：1274-1283.

[2] 白杰，高利利，张志勤，等.电子舌技术的原理及在中药领域的应用[J].中南药学，2021，19（01）：78-84.

[3] 毕胜，谢若男，金传山，等.基于仿生技术的制川乌炮制过程变化研究[J].中草药，2020，51（23）：5956-5962.

[4] 丁影.厚朴炮制前后指纹图谱及主要成分含量变化的研究[J].中国药师，2020，23（09）：1745-1750.

[5] 林好，冯娇，陈圻宇，等.基于HPLC多波长法测定两种熟地黄中有效成分的含量及指纹图谱分析[J].中国食品添加剂，2020，31（11）：94-102.

[6] 李喆，刘博男，张超，等.多指标综合评价结合层次分析法优化酸枣仁炒制工艺[J].中成药，2020，42（08）：2089-2094.

[7] 杨冰，宁汝曦，秦昆明，等.中药材产地加工与炮制一体化技术探讨[J].世界中医药，2020，15（15）：2205-2209+2215.

[8] 刘晓梅，张存艳，刘红梅，等.基于电子鼻和HS-GC-MS研究地龙腥

味物质基础和炮制矫味原理［J］.中国实验方剂学杂志，2020，26（12）：154-161.

［9］贾萌，赵华聪，蔡淑慧，等.HPLC指纹图谱及多成分定量的独活饮片质量评价研究［J］.南京中医药大学学报，2020，36（01）：88-93.

［10］辛二旦，司昕蕾，边甜甜，等.基于响应面法的大黄产地加工炮制一体化工艺研究［J］.中国中医药信息杂志，2020，27（05）：53-57.

［11］吴情梅，刘晓芬，连艳，等.产地加工炮制一体化对川芎饮片化学成分的影响研究［J］.中国药房，2020，31（06）：686-691.

［12］吴情梅，刘晓芬，连艳，等.川芎产地加工与饮片炮制一体化工艺研究［J］.中草药，2019，50（16）：3808-3814.

［13］吴潍.产地初加工方法对中药材质量的影响［J］.中医药管理杂志，2020，28（01）：90-94.

［14］冷晓红，陈海燕，郭鸿雁.电子鼻技术在中药领域的应用［J］.西北药学杂志，2019，34（03）：426-428.

［15］张美龄.荆芥炭止血物质基础及其作用机制的研究［D］.北京：北京

中医药大学，2018.

[16] 吴喆，张霁，左智天，等.红外光谱结合化学计量学快速鉴别云南重楼不同炮制品［J］.光谱学与光谱分析，2018，38（04）：1101-1106.

[17] 黄永亮，余志杰，黎江华，等.熟三七饮片HPLC指纹图谱的建立及多成分定量测定［J］.中草药，2018，49（03）：589-595.

[18] 孙冬月，王晓婷，王馨雅，等.香薷传统切制与产地加工炮制一体化比较研究［J］.中国中医药信息杂志，2017，24（12）：72-76.

[19] 解达帅.基于智能感官技术和模式识别的中药炮制"火候"的研究［D］.成都：成都中医药大学，2017.

[20] 方毅.茯苓产地加工与炮制一体化研究［D］.合肥：安徽中医药大学，2017.

[21] 席啸虎，王世伟，仝立国，等.山药产地初加工及炮制工艺研究［J］.时珍国医国药，2017，28（03）：613-616.

[22] 赵志浩.基于生物效价检测的附子毒效物质辨识与质量控制［D］.承德：承德医学院，2017.

[23] 付智慧,李淑军,胡慧华,等.基于电子舌技术的豨莶草炮制前后滋味比较[J].中草药,2017,48(04):673-680.

[24] 张丽,丁安伟.中药材产地加工-饮片炮制一体化研究思路探讨[J].江苏中医药,2016,48(09):70-71+74.

[25] 杨冰月,李敏,吴发明,等.基于止咳效价评价半夏及其炮制品品质的方法研究[J].中草药,2015,46(17):2586-2592.

[26] 孔铭,白映佳,徐金娣,等.白芍初加工方法和质量控制研究进展[J].世界科学技术-中医药现代化,2014,16(10):2248-2254.

[27] 徐志伟,曹岗,杜伟锋,等.多指标综合评价麸炒白芍的炮制工艺[J].中草药,2014,45(13):1867-1870.

[28] 杨冰月.基于物质基础和生物活性对半夏及其炮制品功效的相关性研究[D].成都:成都中医药大学,2014.

[29] 陈雯雯.苍术麸炒前后氯仿和挥发油部位药效学及化学成分对比研究[D].武汉:湖北中医药大学,2013.

[30] 李会芳,王伽伯,肖小河.基于致泻效价检测的大黄不同炮制品的生物品质研究[J].时珍国医国药,2012,23(05):1215-1216.

[31] 余金喜,马梅芳,刘成亮.葶苈子微波炮制品药效学实验研究[J].中国实用医药,2010,5(27):131-133.

[32] 乌兰其其格,那生桑.草乌炮制品的药理毒理及药效学实验研究[J].内蒙古医学院学报,2009,31(05):482-486.

[33] 曹艳.甘遂醋炙降毒的机理及抗癌活性部位筛选的初步研究[D].武汉:湖北中医药大学,2010.